THE
OPTIMUM
NUTRITION
COOKBOOK

Other books by Patrick Holford

100% Health
500 Top Health and Nutrition Questions Answered
Balance Your Hormones
Beat Stress and Fatigue
Boost Your Immune System (with Jennifer Meek)
Food GLorious Food (with Fiona McDonald Joyce)
Hidden Food Allergies (with Dr James Braly)
How To Quit Without Feeling S**t (with David Miller and Dr James Braly)
Improve Your Digestion
Natural Chill Highs
Natural Energy Highs
Natural Highs (with Dr Hyla Cass)
Optimum Nutrition Before, During and After Pregnancy (with Susannah Lawson)
Optimum Nutrition for the Mind
Optimum Nutrition for Your Child (with Deborah Colson)
Optimum Nutrition Made Easy
Say No to Arthritis
Say No to Cancer
Say No to Heart Disease
Six Weeks to Superhealth
Smart Food for Smart Kids (with Fiona McDonald Joyce)
Solve Your Skin Problems (with Natalie Savona)
The 9-Day Liver Detox (with Fiona McDonald Joyce)
The Alzheimer's Prevention Plan (with Shane Heaton and Deborah Colson)
The Feel Good Factor
The H Factor (with Dr James Braly)
The Little Book of Optimum Nutrition
The Low-GL Diet Counter
The Low-GL Diet Cookbook (with Fiona McDonald Joyce)
The Low-GL Diet Bible
The Optimum Nutrition Bible
The 10 Secrets of 100% Healthy People

Judy Ridgway is an international olive oil expert and the author of more than 60 books on food and wine. She specialises in all aspects of taste and flavour, running seminars and tasting sessions. She also contributes articles to a range of general interest and specialist food magazines. Her website is at www.oliveoil.org.uk

patrick HOLFORD
& Judy Ridgway

THE
OPTIMUM
NUTRITION
COOKBOOK

piatkus

PIATKUS

HB first published in Great Britain in 1999 by Piatkus Books
PB first published in Great Britain in 2000 by Piatkus Books

Reprinted 8 times
This edition published 2010
Reprinted 2010, 2011

A CIP catalogue record for this book
is available from the British Library.

ISBN 978-0-7499-5344-7

Design by Paul Saunders
Photography by Philip Webb

Scanning data capture and manipulation by Wyvern 21 Ltd, Bristol

Printed and bound by L.E.G.O. S.p.A.

Piatkus
An imprint of
Little, Brown Book Group
100 Victoria Embankment
London EC4Y 0DY

An Hachette UK Company
www.hachette.co.uk
www.piatkus.co.uk

Contents

Eat Yourself to Health 7

Acknowledgements

This book would not have been possible without the help and support of many people. A very special thank you goes to Natalie Savona for her help with the editing and to Rachel Winning, our editor at Piatkus, and all her very professional and supportive team.

We are indebted to the many nutritionists who sent in their favourite recipes to help us compile *The Optimum Nutrition Cookbook*. These are: Adri Bester, Charlotte Bridge, Richard Brown, Sally Child, Kay Cruse, Elaine Elliott, Eve Gilmore, Gillian Key, Lorna Marchant, Conner Middelmann-Whitney, Linda Perkins, Natalie Savona, Hilda Solomons, Liz Thearle and Gill Williams – many thanks. Our thanks also go to Anton Mosimann, Lesley Waters, Ursula Ferrigno and Joanna Kjaer. Also to Peter Vaughan and Barney Wan for their recipes.

Guide to abbreviations and measures

1 pound (lb) = 16 ounces (oz)   2.2lb = 1 kilogram (kg)

1 pint = 0.6 litres   1.76 pints = 1 litre

2 teaspoons (tsp) = 1 dessertspoon (dsp)

1.5 dessertspoons = 1 tablespoon (tbsp)

In this book, calories means kilocalories (kcal)

References and further sources of information

Supporting research for statements made in the first part of this book is available from the Lamberts Library at the Institute for Optimum Nutrition (ION) (see page 220), whose members are free to visit and study there. ION also offers information services, including literature and library search facilities, for readers who would like to access scientific literature on specific subjects. A detailed explanation of many of the nutritional principles behind the recipes in this book can be found in my book, *The Optimum Nutrition Bible* (Piatkus).

eat yourself
to health

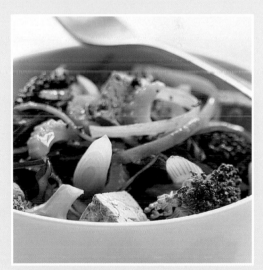

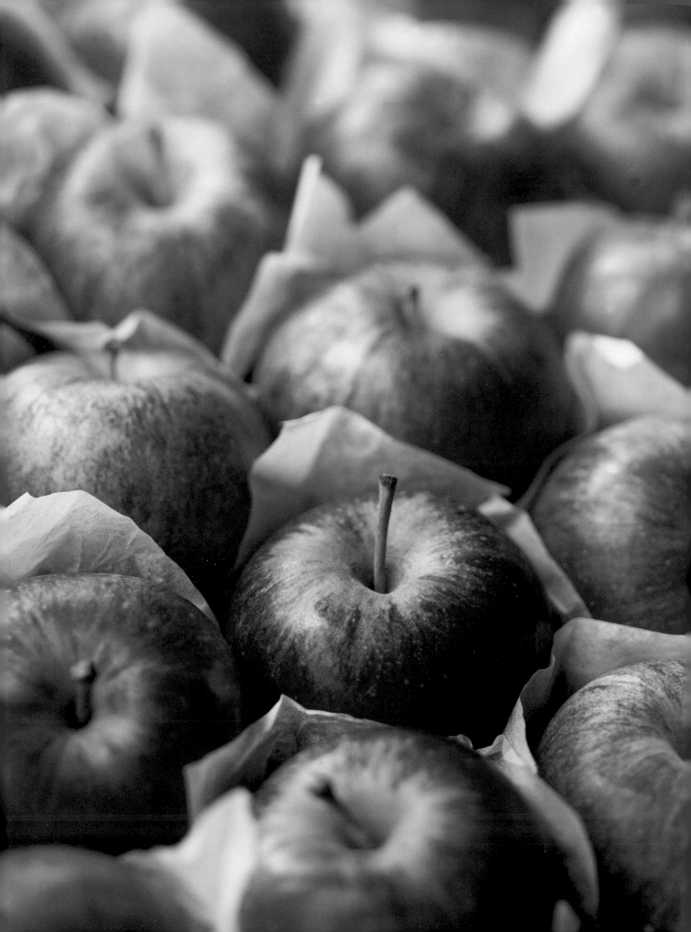

What is Optimum Nutrition?

You *can* have your cake and eat it. You can eat delicious food, great snacks, delightful dinners and desserts *and* enhance your health. So, why not do it? The purpose of this book is to combine 'what tastes good' with 'what does you good' in a straightforward way that you can easily put into practice.

Optimum nutrition simply means giving your body the best possible intake of nutrients to allow it to be as healthy as possible and to work as well as it can. This is a subject I've been researching since 1980 and, together with colleagues at the Institute for Optimum Nutrition, since 1984. We have learnt that being optimally nourished can:

- improve your clarity and concentration
- increase your IQ
- enhance your physical performance
- improve your quality of sleep
- increase your resistance to infection
- protect you from disease
- slow down the ageing process
- more than halve your risk of cancer, heart disease, diabetes and arthritis

These might sound like bold claims, yet each has been proven by proper scientific research. Change what you eat and you not only change your health but also your day-to-day vitality. You add life to your years and years to your life.

If you could achieve all this by eating food that tastes great wouldn't you do it? Of course – and that is what this cookbook is all about. The following pages explain what you need to eat, and how you need to store, prepare and cook food to keep its nutrient content to the maximum. You'll also want to know how to achieve optimum nutrition if you're a vegan, vegetarian or fishitarian or are on a restricted diet, perhaps because of allergies. The recipe chapters put all these principles into practice, giving you a delicious collection of mouthwatering recipes to choose from.

What's in Your Food?

We know that every morsel of food provides dozens of active ingredients that can promote or damage your health. The most important of these ingredients are the essential ones – the ones you need to survive and be healthy. These nutrients include:

- water
- carbohydrate
- protein
- essential fats
- vitamins
- minerals

MACRONUTRIENTS

MICRONUTRIENTS

Water, carbohydrates, protein and essential fats are classified as 'macronutrients' because we need to eat a lot of them. We need vitamins and minerals in relatively smaller amounts, so they are called the 'micronutrients'.

Vitamins in Food

Although vitamins are needed in much smaller amounts than fat, protein or carbohydrate, they are no less important. They switch on enzymes, which in turn make all our body processes happen.

Vitamins are needed to balance hormones, produce energy, boost the immune system, make healthy skin, protect the arteries, and keep the brain and nervous system (and just about every other part of the body) working well.

Minerals in Food

Minerals, like vitamins, are essential for just about every bodily process. Calcium, magnesium and phosphorus help build our bones and teeth. Nerve signals (vital for communication between the brain and muscles) depend on calcium, magnesium, sodium and potassium. Oxygen is carried in the blood by an iron compound. Chromium helps control blood sugar levels. Zinc is vital for all physical repair, renewal and development. Selenium and zinc help boost the immune system. Brain function depends on adequate magnesium, manganese, zinc and other essential minerals. These are only a few of the thousands of key roles minerals play in human health.

In addition to vitamins and minerals, there are hundreds of other, not strictly essential, but health-promoting factors in food, often called phytonutrients (*phyto* = plant). The antioxidants and anti-inflammatory agents found in berries are examples of these.

Knowing What You're Eating

Achieving an optimal intake of each of the vitamins and minerals is a big step towards being super-healthy. Of course, the big question is: how do you know if what you're eating meets your needs? Many people assume it does, but surveys consistently show that the vast majority of us don't even achieve the very basic Recommended Daily Allowance (RDA) levels of nutrients.

- Fruits and vegetables provide most of your vitamins and minerals (except vitamins D and B12).
- Meat, fish, eggs and dairy products provide vitamin D and B12, among other nutrients.
- Dairy products are good for calcium, but poor for other minerals.
- Seeds and nuts are great sources of minerals (and essential fats).
- Processed and refined foods are very low in nutrients.
- 'Living' food has much higher nutrient levels than dried food such as rice.

To achieve an optimal intake of vitamins from food you need to be eating three or more servings of dark green, leafy and root vegetables, and three or more servings of fresh fruit, plus some nuts or seeds every day. Foods especially rich in minerals include kale, cabbage, root vegetables, low-fat dairy produce (such as yoghurt), seeds or nuts such as almonds, as well as fresh fruit, vegetables and wholefoods such as lentils, beans and wholegrains.

These are the micronutrients you need in your diet, but what about getting the right balance of the macronutrients fat, protein and carbohydrate?

Nutritional Supplements

Even if you eat all the right foods you are unlikely to achieve an optimal intake of all vitamins and minerals. The reasons for this, and the benefits that can be obtained from eating the right diet *and* taking nutritional supplements are fully explained in *The Optimum Nutrition Bible* (Piatkus), which also shows you how to work out your own ideal supplement programme.

Although nutritional needs differ from person to person, everyone should take a good multivitamin and multimineral supplement and additional vitamin C each day, providing, at least, the following quantities of vitamins and minerals:

A multivitamin containing at least the following:

vitamin A	2250 µg
vitamin D	10 µg
vitamin E	100 mg
vitamin B1	25 mg
B2	25 mg
B3 (niacin)	50 mg
B5 (pantothenic acid)	50 mg
B6	50 mg
B12	5 µg
folic acid	50 µg
biotin	50 µg

A multimineral containing at least the following:

calcium	150 mg
magnesium	75 mg
iron	10 mg
zinc	10 mg
manganese	2.5 mg
chromium	50 µg
selenium	25 µg

A vitamin C supplement providing 1000 mg vitamin C

Defining the Perfect Diet

For the past 12 years we've been researching the perfect diet. Our conclusions to date are shown in the Perfect Diet Pyramid (see page 14). While, for many, this diet is not going to be achievable overnight, it does give a clear indication of where you should be heading. The general daily guidelines appear at the end of each section.

Fat

There are two main kinds: saturated (hard) fat and unsaturated fat. Saturated fat is not essential – we should eat it seldom if at all. The main sources are meat and dairy products. There are also two kinds of unsaturated fats: monounsaturated fats, high in olive oil; and polyunsaturated fats, found in nut and seed oils, and fish. Certain polyunsaturated fats are essential. These are called linoleic and linolenic acid; they are vital for the brain and nervous system, immune system, cardiovascular system and skin. A common sign of deficiency is dry skin.

The optimal diet provides a balance of these essential fats, also known as Omega 3 and Omega 6 oils. Pumpkin and flax seeds are rich in linolenic acid (Omega 3), while sesame and sunflower seeds are rich in linoleic acid (Omega 6). These essential fats are easily destroyed by heating or exposure to oxygen, so having a fresh daily source is important.

Processed foods often contain hardened or 'hydrogenated' polyunsaturated fats. These are unhealthy and best avoided.

- **Eat** 1 tablespoon cold-pressed seed oil (sesame, sunflower, pumpkin, flax seed, etc.) or 1 heaped tablespoon ground seeds each day.

- **Avoid** fried food, burnt or browned fat, saturated and 'hydrogenated' fat.

Protein

Protein is made out of amino acids, which are the building blocks of the body. As well as being vital for growth and the repair of body tissue, they are used to make hormones, enzymes, antibodies and neurotransmitters, and help transport substances around the body. Both the quality of the protein you eat (determined by the balance of these amino acids), and the quantity, are important.

The best-quality protein foods, in terms of amino acid balance, include eggs, quinoa (a grain that cooks like rice), soya, meat, fish, beans and lentils. Animal protein sources tend to contain a lot of undesirable saturated fat. Vegetable protein sources tend to contain more beneficial complex carbohydrates than meat. It is best to limit your meat intake to three times a week. Many vegetables, especially 'seed' foods like runner beans, peas and broccoli, contain good levels of protein. They also help to neutralise excess acidity which can lead to loss of minerals including calcium – hence the higher risk of osteoporosis among frequent meat-eaters.

- **Eat** three servings of beans, lentils, quinoa, tofu (soya), 'seed' vegetables or other vegetable protein. Occasionally replace with fish, cheese, a free-range egg or lean meat.

- **Avoid** excess animal source protein.

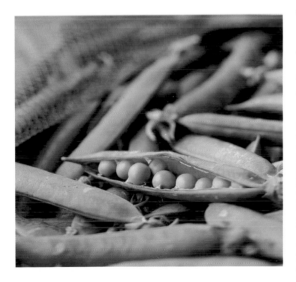

Carbohydrate

Carbohydrate is the body's main fuel. It comes in two forms: 'fast-releasing' (as in sugar, honey, malt, sweets and most refined foods); and 'slow-releasing' (as in wholegrains, vegetables and fresh fruit). The latter foods contain more complex carbohydrate and more fibre, both of which help to slow down the release of sugar.

Fast-releasing carbohydrates are best avoided. Constant use of fast-releasing carbohydrates can give rise to complex symptoms and health problems. Some fruits like bananas, dates and raisins contain faster-releasing sugars and are best kept to a minimum by people with glucose-related health problems. Slow-releasing carbohydrates – fresh fruit, vegetables, pulses and wholegrains – should make up about two-thirds of your diet, or around 65 per cent of your total calorie intake.

Eating these kinds of foods in such quantities will also give you at least 35g fibre which is an ideal daily intake. Fibre absorbs water in the digestive tract, making the food contents bulkier and easier to pass through the body, preventing constipation and the putrefaction of foods. This also slows down the absorption of sugar into the blood, helping to maintain good energy levels.

- **Eat** three or more servings of dark green, leafy and root **vegetables**, such as watercress, carrots, sweet potatoes, broccoli, Brussels sprouts, spinach, green beans or peppers, raw or lightly cooked.

- **Eat** three or more servings of **fresh fruit**, such as apples, pears, bananas (not more than one a day), berries, melon or citrus fruit.

- **Eat** four or more servings of **wholegrains**, such as brown rice, millet, rye, oats, wholewheat, corn, quinoa, pasta or pulses.

- **Avoid** any form of sugar, foods with added sugar, and white or refined foods.

The Perfect Diet Pyramid

Fat
1 heaped tablespoon ground seeds or 1 tablespoon cold-pressed seed oil.

Protein
3 servings beans, lentils, quinoa, tofu (soya) or 'seed' vegetables. Occasionally replace one of these with a small helping of fish, cheese, a free-range egg or lean meat.

Complex Carbohydrates
4 servings of wholegrains, such as brown rice, millet, rye, oats, wholewheat, corn, quinoa, bread or pasta.

Fruit and vegetables
6 servings of fruit and vegetables. Eat citrus fruits, apples, pears, berries and melons. The best vegetables are dark green, leafy and root vegetables.

Top five diet tips

What this all boils down to is five simple guidelines for healthy eating. Every day make sure you eat:

- 1 heaped tablespoon ground seeds or 1 tablespoon cold-pressed seed oil.

- 3 servings beans, lentils, quinoa, tofu (soya) or 'seed' vegetables. If you like, you can occasionally replace one of these with a small helping of fish or cheese, a free-range egg or lean meat.

- 3 pieces of fresh fruit, such as apples, pears, berries, melon or citrus fruit.

- 3 servings of dark green, leafy and root vegetables such as watercress, carrots, sweet potatoes, broccoli, spinach, green beans, peas and peppers.

- 4 servings of wholegrains, such as brown rice, millet, rye, oats, wholewheat, corn, quinoa, bread or pasta.

Balancing Your Diet

Now that you know what it officially means to eat a well-balanced diet, how do you know if you're achieving it?

Based on The Perfect Diet Pyramid, on page 14, a perfect daily diet consists of:

1 serving of essential fats

3 servings of protein

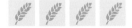

4 servings of complex carbohydrate foods

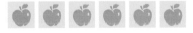

6 servings of fruit and vegetables

In practice, this means:

- 1 heaped tablespoon ground seeds or 1 tablespoon cold-pressed seed oil
- 3 servings beans, lentils, quinoa, fish, tofu (soya), or 'seed' vegetables
- 4 servings of wholegrains, such as brown rice, millet, rye, oats, wholewheat, corn, quinoa, bread or pasta

- 6 servings of fresh fruit, such as apples, pears, bananas (not more than one), berries, melon or citrus fruit and dark green, leafy and root vegetables, such as watercress, carrots, sweet potatoes, broccoli, spinach, green beans, peas and peppers

Each recipe in this book shows you at a glance how many servings of each of these food groups it provides per person. So, for example, if you were to start your day with Simple Fruit Muesli (page 45), you'll get one serving of fruit, one serving of complex carboydrate and one serving of essential fats.

If you were to snack on an apple, then eat Sweet Potato and Carrot Soup (page 109) for lunch, and Red Mullet (see page 188) with steamed broccoli for dinner this is what you would have achieved in a day. (Please note that if you add a piece of fruit, such as an apple, or a serving of vegetable, such as the broccoli, add a to your day's score.)

Simple Fruit Muesli

Sweet Potato and Carrot Soup

Red Mullet with steamed broccoli

apple

You have just had a perfect day, as far as balance of nutrient content is concerned. Of course, no one wants to be doing even this simple equation every day. However, by applying this method of analysing what you eat for a couple of weeks, you'll soon develop an instinct as to what balance of foods you require for optimal health.

Remember though, that many of the serving ratings are quite roughly calculated and rounded up or down, so use them as a general guide only. As long as you are balancing out your meals well over the course of a week, you don't need to reach the exact totals every single day.

The When and How of Eating

It isn't just what you eat that counts, but how and when you eat it. Here are five tips that will help you get more goodness out of your food.

1 Graze, don't gorge

Studies have consistently shown that people who eat little and often are healthier than those who just eat one or two large meals a day. In practice, for most people this means having breakfast, lunch and dinner plus a couple of snacks or fruit in between.

2 Breakfast like a king, lunch like a prince, dine like a pauper

There's a lot of truth to this old saying, with a little modification. Firstly, you need food for energy during the day. So it doesn't make sense to eat half your day's food in the evening. Also, it is definitely not a good idea to go to bed still digesting your dinner. As a general rule, you should eat dinner early and leave at least two hours before going to sleep.

3 Chew your food thoroughly

Chewing your food and eating at regular times really helps you to digest and get the most out of your food.

4 Eat something raw with every meal

The healthiest diet has a large proportion of raw or very lightly cooked food.

5 Eat fruit as snacks and have desserts as treats

Unlike protein-rich foods, fruit doesn't need to be digested in the stomach and will pass rapidly through the stomach for digestion further on in the digestive tract. If you eat a fruit salad after a piece of chicken the fruit will therefore have to stay in the stomach longer than it needs to and may ferment. For this reason, it is generally better not to have fruit or a fruit-based dessert immediately following a protein-rich main course or, at least, have a good break between courses.

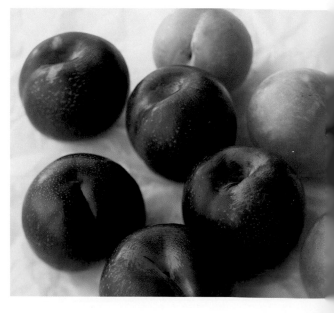

Why Drinking is Good for You

wo-thirds of your body is made up of water, which is therefore the most important nutrient. While you could probably survive without food for up to a month, you'd be dead within three days without water. The body loses 1.5 litres (2½ pints) of water a day, through the skin, lungs, digestive tract and via the kidneys as urine, ensuring that toxic substances are eliminated from the body. We also make about 0.3 litres (0.07 pints) of water a day when glucose is 'burnt' for energy. Therefore, the minimum water intake from food and drink is more than 1 litre (1¾ pints) a day. The ideal intake is around 2 litres a day.

If you don't take in enough water, toxins in the blood and urine become more concentrated and potentially do you more harm by putting a strain on your body's detoxification potential. As part of your optimum diet make sure you take in around 1 litre (1¾ pints) of water a day, taken as pure water or in diluted juices, or herb and fruit teas.

Dilute Fruit Juices

Although fruit juice consists mainly of water, not all of this counts. This is because when your blood sugar level rises, as a result of drinking the sugars in the fruit juice, your body demands more fluid to dilute the sugar in your blood. If, however, you dilute fruit juice with as much water as juice, you supply your body with both energy and fluid. Choose sugar-free juice without additives; the best ones are apple and pear because they contain more slow-releasing sugars.

Tea and Coffee Don't Count

The stimulants in tea and coffee act as diuretics (causing your body to lose water), as well as robbing you of valuable minerals. So they are not recommended as sources of fluid intake. Nor is a lot of tea or coffee good for your health or energy.

Alcohol Dehydrates You

Likewise, alcohol is a diuretic, i.e. it makes the body lose water so it dehydrates you. Probably the healthiest recommendation is not to drink at all, or to limit your intake to three or four drinks a week (preferably red wine). Using small amounts of red wine in cooking is also fine, especially since much of the alcohol tends to boil off. When drinking alcohol it is best to drink some water with it, to prevent dehydration. See the Drinks section on page 211 for plenty of delicious alternatives that are good for you.

Eating for Energy

The foods you eat are the biggest single factor affecting your energy levels. In fact, changing your diet can noticeably boost your energy in as little as 14 days. The reason for this is that the energy that powers your brain, nerves, muscles and indeed every function of your body, is derived from food. The fuel is glucose, a kind of sugar found in carbohydrate foods. However, just eating glucose would be a very bad idea – for two reasons. Firstly, to release the energy from glucose you need a whole lot of vitamins and minerals. These are not present in glucose but *are* present in whole foods. Secondly, glucose is like rocket fuel – you get a rush of energy and then burn out.

The body's favourite fuel is complex carbohydrates, which are more complex sugars that take longer to be broken down into glucose. Examples are oats, rye bread and wholewheat pasta. These are all classified in the chart opposite as having a low 'Glycemic Index' score. This means they release their carbohydrate slowly into the bloodstream, thus making energy available to the body over a longer period of time. This contrasts with sugar (or glucose) which gives a short, sharp boost to blood sugar levels, followed by a dip.

Food Combining

Whether a food is fast- or slow-releasing depends on more than just the type of sugar it contains. The presence of certain kinds of fibre slows down the release of sugars, so whole foods are much better for you than refined foods. It is therefore better to eat brown rice, wholegrain bread and wholewheat pasta rather than the white stuff. This also means that fresh fruit, which contains fibre, is better than fruit juice. The presence of protein in a food also lowers its glycemic index – one reason why beans and lentils, both high in protein and fibre, have such a low GI score. Combining protein-rich foods with slow-releasing carbohydrates (for example, eating fish with rice or chicken with pasta), further helps to even out blood sugar levels.

Generally, foods with a GI score below 50 are great to include in your diet, while those with a score above 70 should be avoided or mixed with a low-scoring food or protein. Those with a score between 50 and 70 should be eaten infrequently and only with a low-scoring food. For example, bananas are quite high, with a score of 62. Whereas oats and skimmed milk are low, with a score of 49 and 32 respectively. Having a bowl of oats with

The Glycemic Index of Common Foods

Food	Score	Food	Score	Food	Score
Sugars		*Breads and biscuits*		*Dairy products/substitutes*	
Glucose	100	French baguette	95	Tofu ice cream	73
Maltose	100	Rice cake	82	Ice cream (low fat)	50
Honey	87	Puffed wholemeal	81	Yoghurt	36
Sucrose (sugar)	59	crispbread		Skimmed milk	32
Fructose (fruit sugar)	20	Water biscuit	76	Whole milk	27
		Waffles	76		
Fruit		Bagel	72	*Vegetables*	
Watermelon	72	White bread	70	Parsnips (cooked)	97
Pineapple	66	Wholemeal bread	69	Potato (baked)	85
Melon	65	Ryvita	69	Potato (instant)	80
Raisins	64	Crumpet	69	Broad beans	79
Banana	62	Pitta bread	57	Pumpkin (boiled)	75
Apricots (fresh)	57	Sourdough rye bread	57	French fries	75
Kiwi fruit	52	Digestive biscuits	59	Potato (new, boiled)	70
Grapes	46	Rich tea biscuits	55	Beetroot (cooked)	64
Orange	40	Oatmeal biscuits	54	Sweetcorn	59
Apple	39	Wholegrain wheat bread	46	Sweet potato	54
Plum	39	Wholegrain rye bread	41	Peas	51
Pear	38			Carrots (cooked)	49
Apricots (dried)	30	*Cereals*			
Grapefruit	25	Cornflakes	80	*Snacks and drinks*	
Cherries	25	Puffed rice	73	Lucozade	95
		Weetabix	69	Pretzels	83
Grains and grain products		Shredded wheat	67	Jelly beans	80
White rice	72	Muesli	66	Corn chips	72
Brown rice	66	Kellogg's Special K	54	Fanta	68
Taco shells	68	Kellogg's All-Bran	52	Mars Bar	68
Couscous	65	Porridge Oats	49	Squash (diluted)	66
Bran muffin	60			Muesli bar with fruit	65
Pastry	50	*Pulses*		Muesli bar	61
Basmati rice	58	Baked beans	48	Popcorn (low fat)	55
Buckwheat	54	Baked beans (no sugar)	40	Potato crisps	54
Apple muffin	54	Butter beans	36	Orange juice	46
White spaghetti	50	Chickpeas	36	Apple juice	40
Instant noodles	46	Black-eye beans	33	Peanuts	14
Wholemeal spaghetti	42	Haricot beans	31		
Barley	26	Kidney beans	29		
		Lentils	29		
		Soya beans	15		

skimmed milk and half a banana for breakfast would help to keep your blood sugar level on an even keel, while eating cornflakes (scoring 80) with raisins (scoring 64) would not do that so well.

The Best Grains

Some grains are better than others because of the type of carbohydrate they contain. Wheat and corn are high in amylopectin, which makes them fast-releasing; while barley, rye and quinoa are higher in amylose, which makes them slower-releasing. Most rice has a high GI score, due to its high amylopectin content. Basmati rice, however, has more amylose and is therefore slower-releasing. Brown basmati is best. Lentils and soya are also low on the GI scale.

How a food is processed makes a difference too. When wheat is turned into pasta the GI score is low, especially if it is wholemeal. When wheat flour is used to make breads, cakes, biscuits or pastry, the GI score goes up. Therefore wholewheat pasta is good, while refined white bread is bad. The best bread is wholegrain rye bread.

Of the grains, oats are among the best. Whole oats, rolled oats, or oatmeal (as used in oat cakes) all have a low glycemic effect.

The Best Fruit and Veg

Most fruits contain fruit sugar (fructose), which is slow-releasing because it first has to be converted to glucose. Some fruits, however (such as grapes, pineapples, watermelon and bananas), contain not only fructose but varying amounts of fast-releasing glucose. A banana may be fine when you've just climbed a mountain and need instant glucose, but it's certainly not the best daily snack. Half a banana with oats is OK, but oats with chopped apple or pear is better in terms of keeping your blood sugar level even.

Many 'sugar-free' foods use grape juice concentrate as a sweetener. This is akin to using glucose. Some use apple juice concentrate which, being high in fructose, is much better.

Almost all vegetables have a negligible effect on blood sugar levels. Those that are worth cutting back on are potatoes, parsnips and swedes which are generally fast-releasing (boiled new potatoes are slower). Although potato crisps may have a lower score, this is due to the high fat content. The same goes for peanuts.

Vitamin Vitality

You need more than fuel to make energy. Once carbohydrates have been digested into glucose, the energy within each unit of glucose is liberated and made available for the body's use by enzymes that depend on vitamins. The most important are the B vitamins – Vitamin B1, B2, B3, B5, B6, B12, folic acid – vitamin C and some minerals. If you lack these seven essential B vitamins or vitamin C you won't make energy efficiently, however much complex carbohydrate you eat.

So, as well as eating complex carbohydrates, you need to eat vitamin-rich foods. The best all-round source of B vitamins and vitamin C is fresh vegetables – lots of them. Combining vegetables with a complex carbohydrate food is a great way to eat for energy.

The Fats of Life

Some fats are good for you. Indeed, eating the right kind of fat is essential for optimal health. Essential fats reduce the risk of cancer, heart disease, allergies, arthritis, eczema, depression, fatigue, infections and PMS – and improve your brain power. If you are fat-phobic you are depriving yourself of essential health-giving nutrients and increasing your risk of poor health. The same is true if you only eat saturated (hard) fat – from dairy products, meat and most margarines. In fact, unless you go out of your way to eat the right kinds of fat-rich foods, such as seeds, nuts and fish, the chances are you're not getting enough good fat.

Good Fats, Bad Fats

There are two main kinds of fat: saturated and unsaturated (either monounsaturated or polyunsaturated). Saturated and monounsaturated fat are not essential nutrients, although they can be used by the body to make energy. Polyunsaturated fats or oils are essential.

Most authorities now agree that, of our total fat intake, no more than one-third should be saturated (hard) fat, and at least one-third should be polyunsaturated oils, with the remaining third coming from monounsaturated fat. Achieving this means eating less meat and dairy produce, and more fish, seeds and their oils.

Polyunsaturated oils come in two families, known as Omega 3 and Omega 6. We need both to be healthy but are most commonly deficient in Omega 3-rich oils. Fish and flax seeds are the best source of Omega 3 oils, while sunflower and sesame seeds are the best source of Omega 6 oils; pumpkin seeds also provide good levels of both.

Seeds

Seeds are not only full of essential fats, they are also packed with protein, vitamins and minerals. Far from being 'fattening', they are an invaluable source of nutrients.

To achieve an optimal intake of essential fats, you need to eat around a heaped tablespoon of seeds a day. Since you require both Omega 3 and Omega 6 oils, your daily seed intake should include some flax, pumpkin or hemp seeds. In practical terms, an ideal mix would be half flax seeds, with the remaining half made up of sesame, sunflower, hemp and pumpkin seeds. Since some of these seeds are quite tough, you will get more nutrients by grinding them in a coffee grinder and then sprinkling them on your

Which Seeds Provide Which Oils?

Seed	Omega 3	Omega 6
Sesame		• •
Sunflower		• • •
Pumpkin	•	• •
Flax (linseed)	• • •	•
Hemp	• •	• • •
Walnut	•	• •
Wheatgerm	•	• •

morning cereal, or in soups, salads and casseroles. Essential fats are easily oxidised and therefore lose their nutritional value if heated or stored too long, especially if exposed to light. So the best way to protect the oils in seeds is to keep them in a tightly sealed glass jar in the fridge.

Essential Oils

Another way to ensure that you get an ideal intake of essential fats is to use cold-pressed seed oils. The value of these oils is destroyed by high temperatures, so don't fry with them. Instead, use them in salad dressings, or add to savoury dishes just before serving. You could also try seed oil instead of butter on baked potatoes and vegetables. If this is your only source of essential fats you need about 1 level tablespoon a day.

Some companies do special cold-pressed oil blends containing different proportions of flax seed oil and other oils to give you the right balance of Omega 3 and 6 oils. These oil blends, or flax seed oil are the best to use, but don't fry with them and keep them in the fridge to stop them going rancid.

The Benefits of Olive Oil

While olive oil contains no appreciable amounts of the essential Omega 3 oils, it is, on average, made up of 10 per cent Omega 6 fats. Only extra virgin and virgin olive oil are 'cold-pressed' and unrefined. Ordinary olive oil may have similar fatty acid levels to virgin oils (although these may have been altered by processing) but it does not have the same antioxidant properties. This makes unrefined olive oils better for you than refined vegetable oils (like the sunflower oil you can generally buy in the supermarket). Also, while there is a strong association between a high intake of saturated fats (mainly from meat and dairy products) and cardiovascular disease, the reverse is true for olive oil. People in Mediterranean countries whose diet includes olive oil have a lower risk of cardiovascular disease. However this may be partly due to a number of other positive factors in their diet, including a high intake of fruit and vegetables and relatively more fish than meat.

The Power of Fish

Carnivorous fish are especially rich in the most powerful of all Omega 3 oils, known as DHA and EPA. Having a good intake of these is linked with better brain function and memory, and less risk of cancer and heart disease.

The best fish to eat are fish with teeth, such as herring, mackerel, tuna or salmon. If this is your only source of essential fats an optimal intake can probably be achieved by eating three servings of fish a week. Once again, if the fish is fried then some of the essential oils will be destroyed so poaching or baking is better.

Average Omega 3 Content in Fish

Fish (100g/3.5oz, uncooked)	Omega 3s (g)
Mackerel, Atlantic	2.5
Herring, Atlantic	1.7
Tuna, Bluefin	1.2
Salmon, Coho	1.0
Turbot (Flatfish)	0.9
Bass, Striped	0.8
Trout, Rainbow	0.7
Shrimp	0.5
Halibut, Pacific	0.4
Flounder*/Sole	0.2

*Analysis on cooked fish

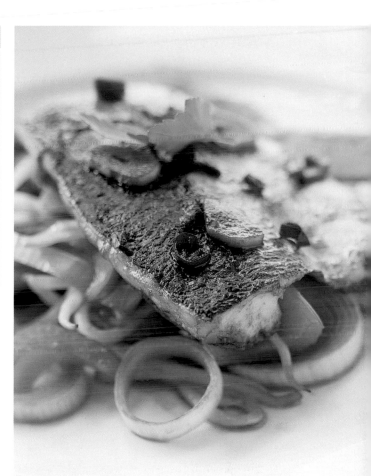

By including in your weekly diet some seeds, some cold-pressed seed oils and some fish it is easy to achieve an optimal intake of essential fats.

Fats to Avoid

Refining and processing vegetable oils can change the nature of the polyunsaturated oil, as in the manufacturing of most margarines. To turn the vegetable oil into a hard fat, the oil is 'hydrogenated'. Although the fat is still technically polyunsaturated the body cannot make use of it. Even worse, it blocks the body's ability to use healthy polyunsaturated oils. This is called a 'trans' fat because it has been changed. Most margarines contain these 'hydrogenated polyunsaturated oils' and are best avoided. So too are foods containing hydrogenated fats, so check the label carefully.

Since hydrogenation is fast becoming perceived as bad for you, some companies now achieve the same goal with a process called 'esterification'. While not as bad as hydrogenation, esterified oils are not as good for you as unrefined, unprocessed, cold-pressed oils. These are best used instead. An example would be to use tahini (sesame spread) or olive oil instead of margarine. The recipes in this book suggest plenty of novel ways to avoid harmful fats and include essential oils in your diet.

Frying is another way to damage otherwise healthy oils. The high temperature makes the oil oxidise; and now, instead of being good for you, oxidised or rancid oils generate harmful 'free radicals' in the body. Frying is therefore best avoided, as is any forming of burning or browning fat.

Anti-Ageing Antioxidants

The oxygen you breathe is your most essential nutrient, yet also the most deadly. You can't make energy without it, but, in the process, harmful oxidants (or free radicals) are produced. These are toxic to the body and need to be disposed of. In fact we receive oxidants from any burning process, be it car exhaust, cigarettes, fried food or strong sunlight. It is this exposure to oxidants that damages cells and increases your risk of getting diseases including cancer, heart disease, Alzheimer's, cataracts, diabetes, arthritis and infections. According to Professor Denham Harman, from the University of Nebraska Medical School, there is a 99 per cent chance that free radicals are the basis for ageing. These oxidants produced by the body every time we turn glucose into energy, eventually kill us. If we take in a lot of oxidants, by smoking or living in a polluted city for example, and consume few antioxidants from fruit and vegetables, we age even more quickly.

Reversing the Ageing Process

The ageing process can be slowed down in three main ways – by decreasing your exposure to oxidants, by increasing your intake of antioxidant nutrients from diet and supplements, and by eating less quantity and more quality foods. Each of these measures has been shown to extend your healthy lifespan. When you eat refined and processed food your body has to work hard to use it up and doesn't get all the nutrients it needs to do the job. So junk food takes more than it gives. On the other hand, if you eat a perfect diet, your body gets exactly what it needs – there are no wasted calories and you don't have to eat so much. By limiting the amount of burnt, browned or fried food you eat, you limit your exposure to oxidants. That's why we recommend other cooking methods, such as steam-frying, poaching, boiling and baking.

Sadly, oxidants are not completely avoidable. There are, however, special nutrients that can mop up oxidants and prevent them from doing their damage. These are antioxidants and one of the most powerful ways in which you can slow down the ageing process is to increase your intake of them.

Foods Rich in Antioxidants

There are many different kinds of antioxidant nutrients, each with their own special role to play in protecting you against the ravages of ageing. Vitamin E protects fat parts of the body, including the essential fats. Vitamin C protects watery parts of the body and makes vitamin E more powerful. Vitamin C is, in turn, protected by glutathione or cysteine found in garlic which, in turn, is protected by anthocyanidins found in berries. Beta-carotene, found in carrots and tomatoes and any red/orange fruit or vegetable, is one of the most important dietary antioxidants.

Overall, if you want to up your intake of antioxidants you need to eat lots of fruit and vegetables, preferably organic, plus fish and seeds. A good guideline is at least five servings of fruit or vegetables a day. Three pieces of fruit, for example, a salad with lunch and a vegetable-based dinner. There are, however, foods that are particularly rich in the key, anti-ageing antioxidant nutrients.

The recipes in this book rely heavily on these antioxidant-rich foods and use methods of preparation that keep their antioxidant power intact.

Detoxifying Foods

Antioxidants don't just protect us from oxidants. There are many other toxic substances that the body has to disarm. These come to us from what we eat and are also generated by the body itself. Much of this detoxification happens in the liver which is one of the largest and most active organs. The chemical processes that turn toxins into substances that can safely be eliminated depend heavily on antioxidants and other nutrients.

Cruciferous vegetables (whose leaves grow in a cross pattern) are especially rich in phytonutrients called isothiocyanates and glucosinolates. These are powerful detoxifying substances and can help break down cancer-causing chemicals. Such vegetables include broccoli, Brussels sprouts, cabbage, cauliflower, cress, horseradish, kale, kohlrabi,

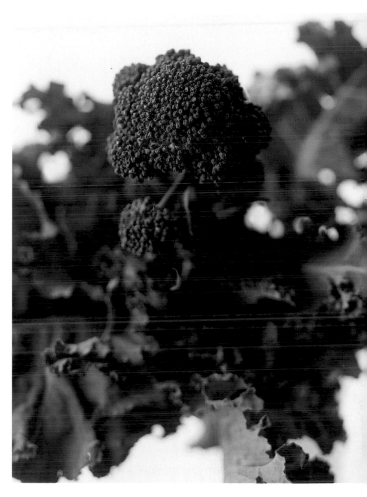

mustard relish and turnip, which have been linked to decreased cancer risk.

Research has shown that if you eat cabbage more than once a week, you are only one-third as likely to develop cancer of the colon as someone who never eats cabbage. In other words, one serving of cabbage a week could cut your chances of cancer of the colon by 60 per cent. Both broccoli and Brussels sprouts have been shown to be protective against cancer – the more you eat, the more protection you get.

Why Colour is Good for You

Multi-coloured plant foods don't just look good on your plate. They *do* you good as well, because each colour relates to different phytonutrients, each with particular health benefits.

Green foods, for instance, are a rich source of chlorophyll and magnesium which is vital for the nerves, muscles and balancing hormones. Yellow foods, such as sweetcorn and yellow peppers, are rich in cartenoids, powerful antioxidants that protect you from cancer.

Mustard and the spice turmeric, the main ingredient in curry powder, are both rich in the pigment curcumin. This is an especially powerful phytonutrient known to fight cancer and to reduce inflammation suffered by people with arthritis.

Orange and red foods often derive their colour from carotenoids such as beta-carotene. Tomatoes and watermelon are rich in another carotenoid called lycopene. These carotenoids are strong antioxidants and help keep you young and healthy. Best sources are foods such as apricots, peaches, melons, watermelon, papaya, mango, carrots and tomatoes.

Beetroot, red grapes and berries derive their red, blue and purple hues from a group of phytonutrients called flavonoids. These are very powerful antioxidants, some of them substantially more powerful than vitamin C. The protective effect of red wine on cardiovascular disease is probably due to these flavonoids. Among the most powerful flavonoids are anthocyanidins which give the purple colour to blueberries, blackberries, blackcurrants and red grapes.

Like the antioxidants, these important phytonutrients each have a different role and work together to keep you healthy. So there are good reasons why colourful food is good for you and why it's a good idea to eat something green, yellow, orange, red and blue every day.

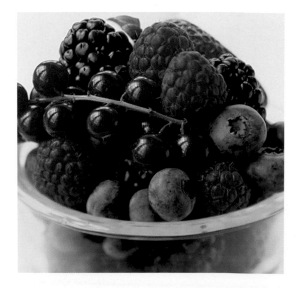

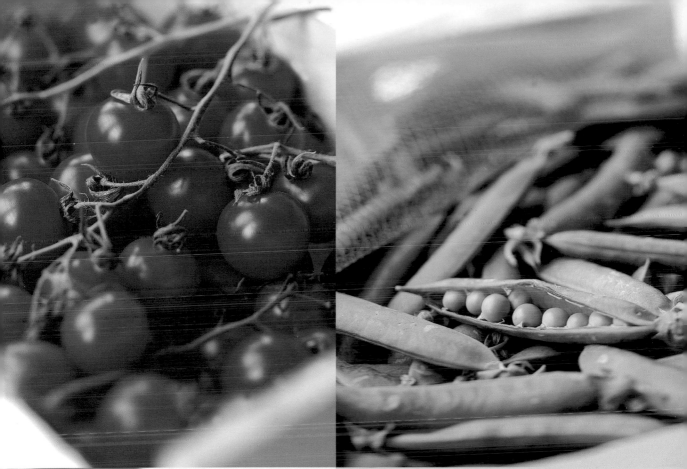
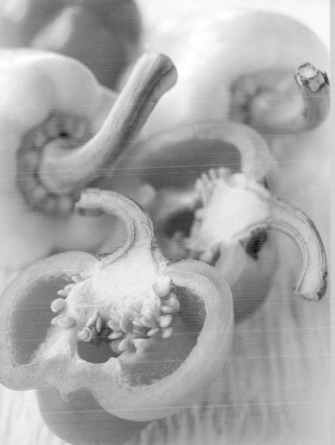

…it's a good idea
to eat something
green, yellow,
orange, red and
blue every day.

Boosting Your Immune System

One of the most powerful immune boosters is vitamin C. It is also a natural anti-viral and anti-bacterial agent. Oranges, while a good source of vitamin C, are by no means the best. The top five foods are carrots, watercress, broccoli, cauliflower and peppers. The top fruits are strawberries and other berries, lemons, then kiwi and other citrus fruit. All these foods contain other phytonutrients that help boost your defences. All in all, perhaps the best vitamin C-rich foods for fighting an infection are blueberries or blackcurrants.

Vitamin A, especially the vegetable form known as beta-carotene, is also vital for maintaining a healthy immune system. Foods rich in beta-carotene are often red or orange in colour, such as carrots and tomatoes.

The Power of Mushrooms

Certain mushrooms are known to boost the immune system and are used as medicine by people with cancer and other immune-related diseases. Among these are shiitake, maitake and reishi mushrooms. Shiitake mushrooms are particularly popular in Japan and are now available in many supermarkets. You can also buy them dry and soak them before cooking. They are an extremely nutritious food and one of the few vegetable sources of vitamin D. Rich in calcium and phosphorus, they also contain high levels of many amino acids including leucine, lysine and threonine, plus the immune-boosting phytochemical, lentinan, a powerful immune stimulant which appears to inhibit virus replication.

Why Garlic Prevents Cancer

Garlic is another important immune-boosting food worth eating on a regular basis. It contains around 200 biologically active compounds, many of which play a role in preventing cancer. By acting as an antioxidant, garlic helps prevent cancer and boosts your immune system.

Garlic contains a compound called allicin which is anti-viral, anti-fungal and anti-bacterial. It's certainly an important ally in fighting infections, and it is wise to include it in your diet. Have a clove a day, and more if you're fighting an infection. As garlic gives viruses, bacteria and parasites a hard time, it's a great food to include in your daily diet when travelling in parts of the world where the risk of picking up a stomach bug is high. Ideally, you should have one or two cloves a day and, when you use it in cooking,

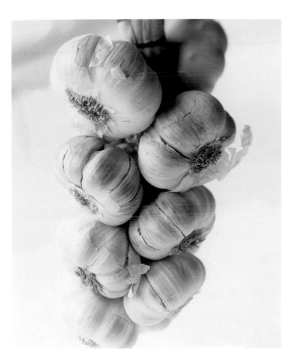

which kills off the bacteria. Only buy 'live' yoghurt, preferably cultured with Lactobacillus acidophilus and or/bulgaricus. These bacteria do not, however, live forever. Depending on how the yoghurt is processed and stored, and when it is eaten, you may get less beneficial bacteria than you think Always keep yoghurt in the fridge and eat it before the 'sell by' date. Once opened, it should be eaten quite quickly.

Feed a Cold, Starve a Fever

If you have an infection, the foods mentioned above are great at keeping you fighting fit. Depending on your state of infection, though, you may need to give your body a rest from digesting foods. Your body is good at telling you this by removing the sensation of hunger – so listen to it. There's a lot of truth in the old saying 'Feed a cold, starve a fever'. Don't eat while you've got a fever and stick to easily digested foods, such as the immune-boosting soups, if you're really fighting a strong infection. However, if you've got a prolonged infection or cold, you'll want to keep your immune strength up.

A number of herbs and spices contain immune-boosting ingredients. Among these are *Uncaria tomentosa*, commonly known as Cat's Claw, a herb native to the Amazon jungle. You can make a delicious tea by boiling up Cat's Claw for five minutes, straining it and adding a dessertspoon of blackcurrant and apple juice concentrate. Ginger and cinnamon are particularly good for sore throats and stomach upsets. Put six slices of ginger in a thermos with a stick of cinnamon and boiling water. Five minutes later you have a delicious, soothing tea. You can add a little lemon and honey too.

don't fry it to death, as that undoes much of the good it can do you.

Yoghurt – The Alternative Antibiotic

Your body contains around 1.5kg (3lb) of bacteria. Most of these are in the digestive tract and are a vital part of your immune defences. These healthy bacteria are capable of making some vitamins; they also help to digest food and prevent disease-causing bacteria or other microbes from taking over. Promoting healthy bacteria is an important part of keeping your body free from infection. And this is where fermented foods, such as yoghurt, can help

Yoghurt is made from milk which is sterilised, then cooled, and 'cultured' by adding live bacteria, which may come from previously prepared yoghurt.

All yoghurts start off containing live bacteria, but long-life or UHT yoghurt is sterilised once it is made,

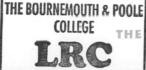

Hormone-Friendly Foods

ormones are chemical messengers that tell the body how to behave. And hormone-like substances abound in natural foods. This is hardly surprising, since hormones are, after all, made from food components. However, the full extent to which certain foods (rich in phytonutrients) influence hormone balance and health has only recently been recognised.

Oestrogen-like plant compounds are often called phyto-oestrogens. Phyto-oestrogens lock onto and block the body's oestrogen receptors, thereby making it harder for harmful chemicals from the environment and the body's own oestrogen, to disrupt hormone signals. These phytonutrients seem to act more like hormone regulators.

Soya and Sex Hormones

One of the best-researched hormone-friendly foods is soya. The soya bean is naturally rich in two isoflavones, called genistein and diadzein, which help to regulate the levels of sex hormones. People who eat soya products on a daily basis and therefore have a high intake of these phytonutrients, have a very low risk of breast cancer and, in men, prostate cancer. An ideal intake for cancer preven-

tion is 100–200mg (4–8fl oz) a day of isoflavones, which is equivalent to a 350g (12oz) serving of soya milk or a serving of tofu. Tofu, a curd made from the soya bean, is the richest source of isoflavones, while very processed soya products are the poorest source. Soya is also an excellent source of protein and should be frequently eaten, in its many different guises, as part of an optimum nutrition diet.

Citrus fruits, wheat, alfalfa, hops, oats, fennel, celery and rhubarb also contain phyto-oestrogens. There is a small amount of evidence that these foods may help to balance hormones and could play a part in helping to reduce symptoms associated with hormonal imbalance. Another food reputed to help balance female hormones is the yam.

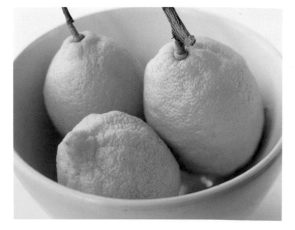

Eating for a Healthy Heart

In almost all cases, heart disease, the major cause of premature death, is completely preventable if you do the right things, which mainly means *eating the right things.* Key prevention foods are fruits and vegetables which are rich in antioxidants such as beta-carotene and vitamin C; fish and seeds, rich in vitamin E and essential fats, and garlic. It's also important to cut down on sugar, saturated fat and salt.

The Fish Factor

As well as providing vitamin E, a powerful antioxidant that can protect fats such as cholesterol from being damaged, fish is a rich source of Omega 3 fats. These essential fats (especially high in herring, mackerel, tuna and salmon) protect against heart disease. This is thought to be the main reason why Japanese people, who generally have a high fish intake, live longer and have less heart disease.

Eating fish three times a week, especially if this is instead of meat (which is high in saturated fat) is a key factor in reducing your risk of heart disease later in life. For vegetarians, the best alternative sources of Omega 3 fats are flax seeds and their oil.

Garlic

Garlic helps prevent heart disease. It lowers cholesterol in the blood and prevents the formation of arterial blockages and clots.

Salt and Blood Pressure

The greater the pressure in the arteries, the narrower they become. And this increases the risk of a stroke, heart attack or thrombosis. Arterial pressure is, to a large extent, controlled by a layer of muscle in the arterial wall. This muscle contracts or expands, depending on the concentration of sodium (salt), potassium, magnesium and calcium in the arteries. While sodium can raise blood pressure and should therefore be restricted in your diet, calcium, magnesium and potassium all lower blood pressure.

Icelandic salt, however, marketed as Solo salt and available in some supermarkets, has more or less equal proportions of sodium and potassium, plus significant quantities of magnesium. It is therefore a healthy alternative to regular salt.

A diet high in fruit, vegetables, nuts, seeds and fish and low in salt, dairy produce and saturated fat can reduce your risk of heart disease.

Choosing, Storing and Preparing Food

There's a saying that 'good food goes off – and the trick is to eat it before it does'. The fresher your food, the greater its nutrient content, and the better it is for you. The foods you choose, and the way you store and prepare them, can make a big difference to what you get from them.

At least half your diet should consist of 'live' food – food that goes off unless you eat it. The difference in the vitamin content of live foods, such as fruit and vegetables, and stored foods, such as rice or beans, is substantial. Even though foods such as brown rice and beans are good sources of complex carbohydrate, protein and minerals, the act of drying and storing them for many months does decrease their vitamin content considerably.

Choose Organic

Raw, organic food is the most natural and beneficial food for the body. In straightforward nutritional analyses, organic food tends to have more in it, both in terms of dry weight and nutrients. The average price difference between organic produce and non-organic produce is around 20 per cent. But organic produce contains, on average, 26 per cent more dry matter, thus actually making it cheaper to buy organic. It is especially important to buy organic grains. Imagine, once each grain has been sprayed, how much you are exposed to.

Genetically Modified Foods

There are many reasons for avoiding genetically modified food. Firstly, most currently available genetically modified (GM) foods, such as soya, are modified to make them resistant to pesticides or herbicides. This means that everything can be sprayed – killing all bugs and weeds, leaving only the soya plant to survive. Such practices generate more yield, higher profit for the farmers, higher profit for the GM seed and herbicide supplier – and a food sprayed in herbicides for the consumer.

The second reason why it's better to avoid GM foods is that they may not be safe. Several trials involving GM food have already been stopped for this reason. Until we can be sure which products contain GM ingredients, it's probably best to avoid all processed foods as many do contain soya derivatives. Some supermarkets will provide a list stating which foods that they stock are non-GM; ask your local store manager.

Choose 'Seed' Foods

Any food that contains the seed from which the next generation of plants will grow, has quite a high nutrient content. This is because the seed has to contain the nutrients necessary for the plant to grow in its early stages, before nutrients are absorbed through the roots. So peas, broad beans, runner beans and corn on the cob are good. Although broccoli is not a seed food, there are plenty of nutrients in its florets (flowers), making it another nutrient-rich vegetable. Stored, dried seed foods, such as beans, lentils, brown rice and wholegrains, also contain significant amounts of minerals, protein and other nutrients.

Freezing and Canning

On the whole, deep-frozen foods keep their nutrient content quite well. There is, for example, little difference in the nutrient content of deep-frozen peas and fresh peas, once boiled.

Canned food is also a reasonably good way of preserving the nutrient content in a food. Some cans, however, have a thin layer of plastic on the inside which can be harmful. So check the inside of your cans and don't live on canned food alone.

Storing Food

Fresh food is best stored in a cool, dark place and eaten relatively quickly. This limits the amount of oxidation, which reduces nutrient content, especially of antioxidants like vitamin C. Chilled foods, kept for two weeks in the supermarket, and one week in your fridge, will have lost a lot of their vitamin vitality. The best thing to do with all food is to buy it and eat it fresh.

Meat, fish and eggs sometimes contain small amounts of various bacteria and, in the case of fish, parasites. For this reason it is very important to buy them fresh, store them for as little time as possible and cook them well before eating. If you store meat or fish in the fridge, make sure it is in a well-sealed container, so that it does not come into contact with other foods. If you do not have the opportunity to buy fresh meat or fish regularly, you could store it in the deep-freeze.

Preparing Food

While it is a good idea to thoroughly scrub or peel non-organic produce to reduce the pesticide and herbicide levels, some people advocate not cleaning organic foods at all. They argue that bacteria in the soil provide vitamin B12 which is lacking in plant foods – however, the manure used to fertilise organic produce is also likely to contain unwanted bacteria, so it is probably best to give it a good wash.

When cleaning non-organic foods, adding a tablespoon of vinegar acidifies the water and may help remove more of the external contaminants. If you are eating a non-organic cabbage or lettuce it is best to throw away the outer leaves as these are likely to be more contaminated. One way of killing unwanted micro-organisms is to put a few potassium permanganate crystals into a sinkful of water, soak the vegetables for a while and rinse them well. Potassium permanganate is available cheaply in most chemists – just ask at the pharmacy counter.

To preserve their nutrient content, cut up fresh foods just before you are about to use them. As soon as a large amount of the surface area inside a plant is exposed to oxygen, nutrient losses are rapid.

Cooking – The Best Methods

More than half the nutrients in the food you eat are destroyed before they reach your plate – depending on the food you choose, how you store it and how you cook it. Every process your food goes through, whether boiling, baking, frying or freezing, takes its toll on vital vitamins and minerals.

It is therefore most desirable to cook foods as little as possible, meaning a shorter time at a lower temperature. The exception here is foods, such as meat and fish, where higher temperatures help kill off micro-organisms if present.

Which Method is Best?

Boiling

This method of cooking causes considerably more losses than steaming. Losses can be kept to a minimum by using as little water as possible, keeping the lid on, and cooking the food as whole as possible. If you do boil vegetables, freeze the water in ice cube trays and use it whenever a recipe calls for stock (e.g. soup) or to cook rice.

Baking

Baking is good, especially if the food is large and has a thick skin (e.g. a pumpkin). Avoid coating food with oil as this increases oxidation. You can roast a potato without adding oil. Losses tend to be less than boiling.

Frying

Keep frying to a minimum, and avoid deep-frying altogether. When you do fry, use butter or coconut oil (saturated fat) or olive oil (monounsaturated) rather than other vegetable oils (polyunsaturated oils), since these are much more prone to oxidation which creates dangerous free radicals.

Grilling

Grilling foods that contain fat is less damaging than frying. However, browning or burning a food does create free radicals. Barbecued food is particularly bad in this respect.

Steam-frying

This involves frying foods with a very small amount of oil and some water, vegetable stock, soya sauce or some other water-based sauce. As soon as a lid is put on, the foods are effectively steamed. The temperature is much lower when you cook using this method so it is all right to use polyunsaturated vegetable oils, such as sesame oil.

Pressure-cooking

Make sure you don't add too much, or too little, water. Pressure-cooking is not that much better than boiling in a small amount of water, and not as good as steaming.

Waterless cooking

This is possible using specially designed pans in which you can 'boil' foods by steaming them in their own juice and 'fry' foods with no oil. These methods are excellent for preserving both nutrient content and flavour.

Microwaving

Relatively smalll amounts of nutrients are lost when microwaving. It is better to use lower settings and longer times. Cover dishes to encourage steaming, although you do need to leave some room for steam to escape.

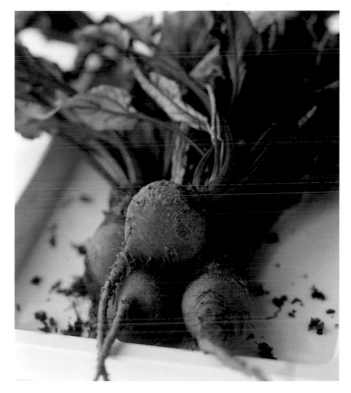

Top ten nutrient tips

- Buy foods as fresh and unprocessed as possible and eat them soon afterwards.

- Keep fresh food in the fridge in sealed containers – cool, covered and in the dark.

- Eat more raw food. Be adventurous. Try raw beetroot and carrot tops in salad, for example.

- Prepare foods cold where possible (e.g. Carrot Soup in the Raw, page 105), and heat to serve.

- Cook foods as whole as possible, slicing or blending before serving.

- Use as little water as possible, preferably steaming.

- Fry foods as infrequently as possible.

- Favour slow-cook methods that use less heat.

- Buy foods cooked by this method (e.g. Scandinavian bread rather than French bread).

- Don't overcook, burn or brown food.

Vegans, Vegetarians and Fishitarians

You don't have to be a vegetarian to be optimally nourished but you can certainly achieve optimum nutrition as a vegetarian. Whichever label applies to you, it is a good idea to increase your intake of vegetable-based foods and reduce or cut out red meat, which is often high in saturated fat. Red meat (unless organic or wild game) is likely to have come from animals which have been treated with antibiotics or hormones, and these can end up in the meat you eat. The first step that people often take is to avoid red meat and become a 'fishichickitarian' (demi-vegetarian) instead – choosing fish or free-range chicken in place of meat.

Fishitarians

The next step for some is to become a fishitarian. This is probably the easiest way to achieve an optimal intake of all nutrients, since fish is a good source of Omega 3 fats that are otherwise quite hard to come by. Omega 3 fats are particularly high in salmon, tuna, herring and mackerel. Eating fish two or three times a week will give you an optimal amount of these nutrients, plus proteins and vitamins B12 and D, neither of which are found in plant foods. For these reasons we have included a number of fish recipes in the following chapters.

However, fish is not without its potential problems. For instance, fish caught in polluted waters retain the pollutants in their flesh, so it is not advisable to eat such fish.

When you choose fish, don't skimp on quality and, whenever possible, choose fish that are likely to come from unpolluted waters and that have not been farmed. Carnivorous fish (those with teeth) are more likely to contain larger amounts of Omega 3 fats. Squid, octopus, shrimps and prawns contain a larger proportion of saturated fat so it is better to limit your intake of these.

Fish should be poached or baked, rather than fried, as these cooking methods are less likely to destroy the essential fats they contain. Smoked fish is also fine. The smoking process involves placing the whole fish on racks, through which heat and woodsmoke pass. The fish cooks slowly; and the flesh inside is not oxidised by the smoke and is therefore not greatly damaged.

Vegetarians

Vegetarians are people who eat plant-based foods plus eggs and dairy produce. Generally speaking, it is considered healthier to be a vegetarian, yet many vegetarians actually eat quite an unhealthy diet because they rely too much on wheat (bread, cereal and pasta) and dairy products (cheese, milk and yoghurt). These two food groups are the two most common food allergens.

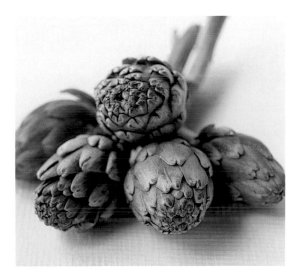

Both eggs and dairy produce are good sources of vitamin B12 and vitamin D, as well as protein. However, a vegetarian need not rely on these as their only source of protein. There is plenty of protein in beans, lentils, seeds, nuts and grains (especially rice, soya and quinoa).

In summary, for a healthy vegetarian diet:

- Don't rely solely on cheese and eggs as sources of protein.
- Include plenty of beans, soya, lentils, seeds and nuts.
- Include wholegrains, such as quinoa, millet and brown rice.

The Best Protein Foods

Quinoa

Quinoa (pronounced 'keenwa'), which has been grown for 5,000 years and is reputed to have given the Aztecs their enormous strength, contains significantly more protein than any grain, and the quality of its protein is better than meat. Quinoa is not technically a grain, but rather a fruit. Nutritionally, it is quite unique, containing more protein than a grain, and more essential fat than fruit. It is also rich in vitamins and minerals, providing almost four times as much calcium as wheat, plus extra iron, B vitamins and vitamin E. Quinoa is also low in fat and the majority of its oil is polyunsaturated, providing essential fatty acids. As such, quinoa is about as close to a perfect food as you can get.

Quinoa can be found in many healthfood stores and may be used as an alternative to rice. To cook it, add twice as much water and boil for 15 minutes.

Soya

Another excellent protein-rich food is soya. The easiest way to eat soya is as 'tofu', which is the curd of the soya bean. Tofu is second only to quinoa in terms of protein quality and is again an excellent source of protein and slow-releasing carbohydrate. Both tofu and quinoa, when eaten with carbohydrate-rich foods, slow down the release of their sugars.

As tofu is the curd of the soya bean it's a bit like a bland cheese. It is available soft (good for desserts or making things 'creamy') or hard (better for steam-fries and main meals). Although it tastes quite bland, tofu absorbs the flavour of any sauce. You can also add flavour to tofu by marinating it for 20 minutes. You can even make a tofu steak or include it in sandwiches. Always drain off the liquid in the packet first.

While quinoa and soya have the right balance of amino acids (the constituents of protein), most vegetable protein is not so complete and is therefore considered inferior in quality to meat protein. You can increase the effective quality of the protein you eat by combining foods from different food groups so that low levels of certain amino acids in one food group are balanced by high levels in another. Eating a varied diet across the different food groups over a 48-hour period, will improve your protein nutrition. Combining rice with lentils, for example, increases the usability of proteins by a third.

Eggs

Eggs are another vegetarian source of protein. However, they are also high in fat, which makes up two-thirds of their calories, and so it is not ideal to eat them on a daily basis. It is best to buy eggs from free-range, grain-fed chickens and not to fry them as the intense heat destroys the essential fats they contain.

Vegans

Some people go one step further and avoid all animal produce, including dairy products and eggs. Again, this can be completely compatible with optimum nutrition – it just means that you need to take more care to get all the right nutrients. The two nutrients lacking in a vegan diet are vitamin B12 and vitamin D. Some bacteria produce vitamin B12, so fermented food can provide a source. Yoghurt, for example, could be made using soya milk, providing B12 made by the bacteria within.

It is probably a lot easier and safer to supplement an all-round multivitamin that provides both vitamin B12 and vitamin D.

Vegans and vegetarians also need to eat seeds (especially flax seeds) to obtain sufficient intake of the Omega 3 essential fats. Flax seeds are by far the richest source of Omega 3 fats, followed by pumpkin seeds and hemp seeds. We recommend a tablespoon a day, preferably ground up and put on cereal, salad or soup, as the grinding helps make the nutrients more available. This is especially important for women who are pregnant or breast-feeding, as the infant relies on Omega 3 fats to build a healthy brain and nervous system.

Vegans also need to make sure they get around 40g protein a day, so it is especially important to eat the equivalent of three to four servings of beans, lentils, quinoa, tofu or seeds. Grains such as rice also contain protein but not as much as beans or lentils. In reality, the best way to achieve the right amount on a vegan diet is to have a good tablespoon of seeds on a grain-based breakfast cereal, plus two main meals that each contain a substantial amount of either beans, lentils, quinoa or tofu.

Two-thirds of the recipes in this book are vegan and hence suitable for vegetarians as well. The small number of recipes that include dairy products (milk, yoghurt and cheese) can easily be converted to vegan recipes by using soya versions of these instead.

> **In summary, for a healthy vegan diet:**
>
> - Include plenty of beans, soya, lentils, seeds and nuts.
>
> - Include wholegrains, such as quinoa, millet and brown rice.
>
> - Take a good multivitamin and multimineral supplement which includes vitamins D and B12.

Allergy-Free Food

An estimated one in two people have adverse reactions to one food or another, most commonly wheat, dairy produce, yeast and sugar. Reactions to sugar are probably not true allergies or intolerances – rather, an indication of a sensitive blood sugar balance, best helped by eating slow-releasing carbohydrates and the kinds of foods included in our recipes, and avoiding sugar.

Wheat-Free food

Allergic reactions to wheat are extremely common and are probably due to the high gluten content of this grain. Gluten is an intestinal irritant and is very hard to digest. Consequently, it is more likely to pass across the lining of a damaged and more permeable digestive tract and into the blood, where the immune system will respond by treating it as an invader. This is an allergic reaction. An extreme version of this is called coeliac disease.

Alternatives include rye, oats and barley, which contain smaller amounts of gluten. Gluten-free grains include rice, millet and quinoa. In practical terms, avoiding wheat means replacing the items on the left of the following chart with some or all of the items on the right.

Instead of . . .	Eat
Wheat bread	100% rye bread (volkornbrot, sonnenbrot, pumpernickel, rye, soda bread, or make your own)
Wheat pasta	100% buckwheat noodles (some times called Soba), rice noodles, or pasta made from corn, quinoa or rice
Wheat cereal	Oat flakes, rye flakes, millet flakes
White sauce	Use cornflour instead of wheat flour

Many of the recipes in this book are wheat-free. For those that aren't, you can use any of the above substitutes.

Dairy-Free Food

Some people who are allergic to cow's milk find they can occasionally tolerate altered forms of cow's milk products such as yoghurt. A greater proportion can tolerate goat's or sheep's milk products. These can easily be substituted in the small number of recipes that include milk, cheese or yoghurt.

For those who are allergic to all forms of dairy produce or who prefer to eat a dairy-free diet, the items on the left of the chart (see following page) can easily be replaced by the items on the right. All are available from health food shops:

Instead of . . .	Eat
Milk	Soya milk, rice milk or oat milk
	On cereal – fruit juice
Cream	Soya cream or cashew cream (see page 201)
Yoghurt	Soya yoghurt, either buy it or make your own (see page 49)
Cheese	Soya 'cheese'
Cream cheese/ Fromage frais	Soft tofu
Butter	Tahini or cold-pressed extra virgin olive oil

Yeast-Free Food

Of all the foods to avoid, yeast is probably the most difficult because it is hidden in many processed foods. Many of the recipes in this book are yeast-free or can easily become so by replacing the items on the left of the chart (below) with those on the right.

Instead of . . .	Eat
Bread with yeast	Oat cakes, rice cakes, original Ryvita, corn tortillas, yeast-free soda bread – or make your own (see pages 46-8)
Beer and wine	Champagne, tequila, vodka (in moderation, of course!)
Vinegar	Lemon juice
Yeasted vegetable stock	Marigold yeast-free stock powder

The more you buy unadulterated food and prepare your own meals, the easier it becomes to devise a varied, delicious and healthy allergy-free diet.

Sugar-Free Food

Sugar is another food that is very hard to avoid as it is added to many processed foods and is often not listed as such. It comes under other names such as glucose, glucose syrup, corn syrup, dextrose and maltose. It's even worth working out how many other sweeteners you eat (such as honey, molasses or dried fruit) because they all have a similar effect on blood sugar (see chapter 6). Use these in moderation. Quite often, sugar-free foods use chemical sweeteners instead. It's much better to buy a plain variety (e.g. of yoghurt) and brighten it up yourself by adding fruit and perhaps a dash of honey. Many of the recipes in this book are sugar-free – they use the natural sweetness of foods to satisfy that desire for a sweet taste that we all have at some time or another. Even some savoury foods, such as cooked carrots, parsnips and lentils, can do this. Once you've weaned yourself off such habits as sugar in tea, you may be surprised how much your tastebuds and cravings change.

Instead of . . .	Eat
Sugar (in baking, teas)	Honey, rice syrup, apple juice
Sugar (on cereals, in yoghurts)	Chopped banana, grated apple
Sugary cereals	Oats, millet, sugar-free varieties
Jams and marmalades	Sugar-free fruit spreads
Chocolate bars	Sugar-free fruit and grain muesli bars, Panda licorice bars, dried fruit
Fruit cordials	Sugar-free fruit drink concentrates

breakfasts

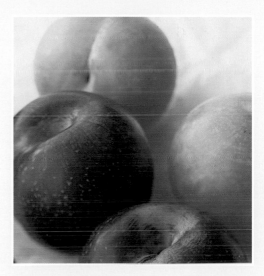

Breakfast is the most important meal of the day since your body's sugar level is at its lowest when you've just woken up. Yet it's all too easy to grab a quick drink and a bowl of cereal or simply a piece of toast.

To fuel your morning activities effectively and keep going until lunchtime, you need a good deal more than this.

The Ultimate Power Breakfast (see below) is the best all-in-one answer. It does not take much preparation and you can eat it day in, day out. However, if you do begin to tire of it, there are plenty of other recipes in this chapter which will give you a good start to the day.

If you want to add to the protein content of your breakfast or to eat a larger first meal of the day, there are more recipes which can be served at the beginning of the day in the chapter on Light Meals (see pages 53-76).

the ultimate power breakfast

Not only does this recipe offer optimum nutrition, it's also a great way to meet your daily five-fruit requirement.

Instead of leaving fruit to go mouldy or mushy in a fruit bowl, the Ultimate Power Breakfast ensures that you get a head start at the beginning of the day. Any additional fruit eaten later on becomes an added bonus!

Here's how to put the Ultimate Power Breakfast together.

method   **1** Blend 250g (9oz) low-fat, organic yoghurt with a variety of fruit in a food processor. Choose four or five fruits from the following:

- **bananas** (we usually include two for carbohydrate content and to make the mixture thick and velvety)

- **kiwis**

- **mangoes**

- **berries** (frozen in winter)

- **pears**

- **apricots, peaches, nectarines, plums**

- **figs**

- **apple sauce** (especially in winter when the choice of fruit diminishes)

- **dried fruit**, soaked and reconstituted overnight (also a good winter choice)

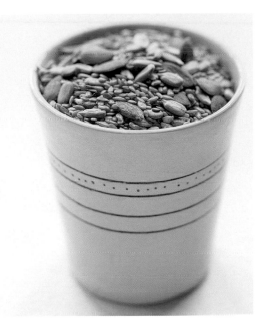

2 Separately, finely grind 4–6 level tablespoons five-seed mix in an electric coffee grinder: flax, sesame, pumpkin, sunflower and hemp. Mix these whole seeds ahead of time and store in the fridge (see page 21 for proportions).

3 Stir the ground seeds into the yoghurt and fruit mix. Then add 2–3 tablespoons cold-pressed mixed seed oil.

4 Blend in a food processor until the mixture has a smooth, creamy texture. Add water or milk if you want to drink it. Otherwise serve in a soup bowl. Enjoy immediately to avoid discoloration and oxidation.

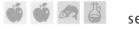 **serves 2**

berry booster

This makes a wonderful start to the day in summer when there are plenty of berries available. Serve on its own or add to your usual muesli or porridge. Choose individual berries or mix and match to get the best flavours.

ingredients
250g (9oz) low-fat natural live yoghurt
225g (8oz) berries (e.g. strawberries, blueberries, raspberries, blackcurrants or blackberries)
2 tablespoons wheatgerm
2 level tablespoons five-seed mix (see above), freshly ground

method **1** Place all the ingredients in a blender and process until smooth. Serve at once.

 **serves 2**

muesli

anton mosimann's oat muesli with fruit

Muesli was invented in Switzerland so it is not surprising that this world-renowned Swiss chef should have come up with the king of muesli recipes. Here it is.

ingredients

2 tablespoons rolled oats
1 dessertspoon oat germ and bran
50ml (2fl oz) warmed skimmed milk
75g (3oz) low-fat natural live yoghurt
2 tablespoons honey
1 tablespoon lemon juice
½ red apple, washed and grated with the skin on
½ green apple, washed and grated with the skin on
2 tablespoons toasted hazelnuts, chopped
150g (5½oz) berries (e.g. strawberries, raspberries, currants and blueberries)
sprigs of mint, to garnish

method

1 Soak the rolled oats and oat germ and bran in the warm milk for at least 2 hours.

2 Stir in the yoghurt, honey and lemon juice. Next, add the freshly grated apples and chopped nuts, and fold into the mixture. Finally, add the berries and decorate with sprigs of mint.

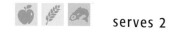 serves 2

mixed cereal muesli with grated apples or pears

You can add variety by using the different kinds of flaked cereals on sale in specialist healthfood and organic shops to make muesli with different tastes and textures. Avoid wheat or rye flakes if you have a problem with gluten.

ingredients   75–100g (3–3½oz) mixed cereal flakes (e.g. wheat, rye, oats, millet, rice)
                 1 tablespoon raisins
                 2 level tablespoons five-seed mix (see page 43), freshly ground
                 2 apples or pears, grated or finely chopped
                 a little lemon juice
                 150g (5½oz) low-fat natural live yoghurt

method   **1** Place the mixed cereal flakes in two soup bowls, add the raisins and 100–125ml (3½–4fl oz) water. Soak the flakes overnight.

2 Sprinkle on the ground seed mix. Grate or chop the fruit and mix with a little lemon juice to prevent discoloration.

3 Spoon the fruit onto the muesli, top with yoghurt and serve at once.

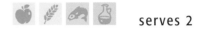   serves 2

simple fruit muesli

If you keep using different fruits you'll never get bored with muesli.

ingredients   75–100g (3–3½oz) oat flakes or porridge oats
                 2 dessertspoons wheatgerm
                 250g (9oz) fruit (e.g. sliced bananas, chopped mangoes or pawpaw, or soft fruit)
                 150g (5½oz) low-fat natural live yoghurt
                 1 heaped tablespoon five-seed mix (see page 43), freshly ground, or mixed chopped almonds and hazelnuts

method   **1** Place the oat flakes or porridge oats in two soup bowls and cover with 100–125ml (3½–4fl oz) water. Leave to soak overnight.

2 Add the wheatgerm and top with the fruit and yoghurt.

3 Sprinkle on the ground seeds or chopped nuts, and serve at once.

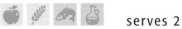   serves 2

bread

tomato scofa bread

*No yeast -— and no waiting – in this really quick and easy bread recipe from Lesley Waters'
Broader Than Beans cookbook. She also suggests an interesting variation with olive oil,
caraway seeds and dill in place of the sun-dried tomatoes, sun-dried tomato oil and chives.*

*The original recipe uses ordinary white flour but you can also make it very successfully
with wholemeal flour but allow a further 3–5 minutes' cooking time.*

ingredients

225g (8oz) plain flour
a pinch of salt
3 level teaspoons baking powder
black pepper (to taste)
4 sun-dried tomatoes in oil, drained and chopped
2 tablespoons freshly chopped chives
about 150ml (5fl oz) milk
2 tablespoons sun-dried tomato oil

method

1 Preheat the oven to 220°C/425°F/Gas 7.

2 Sift the flour, salt and baking powder into a large bowl. Grind in some black pepper. Stir in
the sun-dried tomatoes and chives.

3 Mix the milk and tomato oil together and add to the flour mixture. Gently combine to form
a soft and manageable dough, adding extra milk, if necessary.

4 On a lightly floured surface, roll the dough out to about 2.5cm (1in) thick. Form into a round
about 15cm (6in) in diameter. Score into six triangles with a knife, taking care not to cut all the
way through the dough.

5 Place on a baking tray and bake the bread for 12–15 minutes until risen and golden brown.

1 slice = 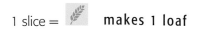 **makes 1 loaf**

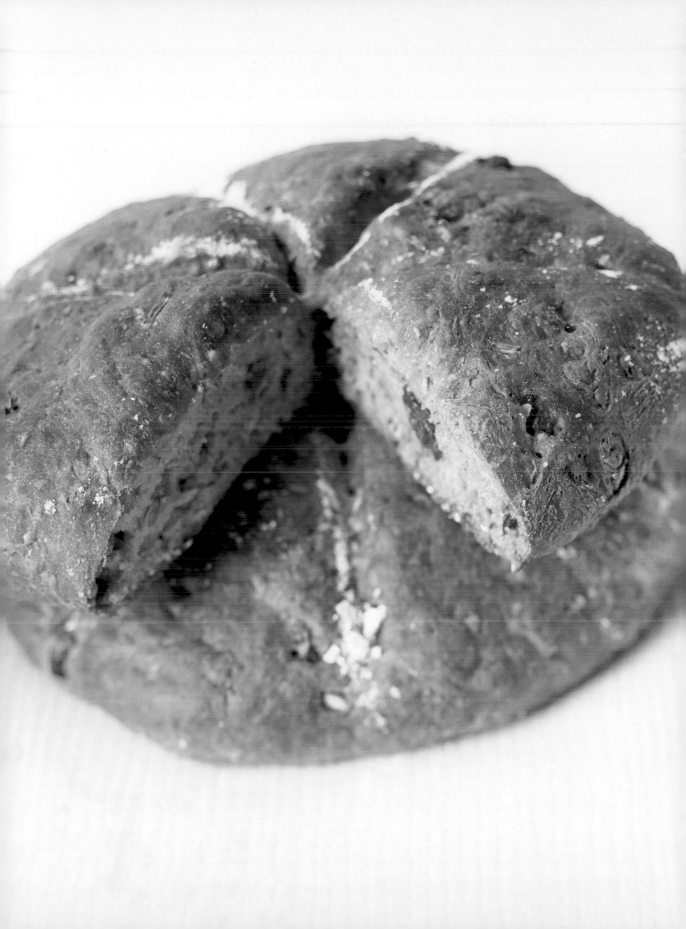

herby corn bread

There is no wheat, yeast or sugar in this quickly prepared bread made from yellow corn-meal. Omit the herbs when you want a plain bread to go with a particular dish. Eat as soon as the bread has cooled or later on the same day.

ingredients

175g (6oz) yellow cornmeal
1½ teaspoons bicarbonate of soda
1 teaspoon mixed dried herbs
¼ teaspoon salt
1 egg
150g (5½oz) low-fat natural live yoghurt
2 tablespoons extra-virgin olive oil

method

1 Set the oven to 200°C/400°F/Gas 6 and grease a 15cm (6in) shallow sandwich tin, muffin pans or bun tray. If using a sandwich tin, line the base with baking parchment.

2 Mix the cornmeal, bicarbonate of soda, herbs and salt in a bowl. Beat the egg separately and mix with the yoghurt and oil. Pour over the dry ingredients and mix well together.

3 Spoon the mixture into the prepared tins and level out. Bake for 15–20 minutes until golden and firm to the touch. Cool on a wire rack and serve.

1 slice = **makes 1 loaf, 6 muffins or about 9 buns**

home-made yoghurt

It is very easy to make yoghurt at home and you can save quite a bit of money by doing so. One way is to invest in an electric yoghurt-maker, which will incubate the yoghurt at the correct temperature, but you can use a wide-neck thermos flask instead.

The type of milk you choose is important. Anything other than UHT or long-life milk must be boiled and cooled before use to reduce the risk of harmful bacteria growing in the incubating yoghurt.

You can make yoghurt with skimmed, semi-skimmed or full-fat milk. If you are using skimmed milk, you may like to add 1–2 tablespoons non-fat dried milk powder to give the yoghurt more body.

ingredients

600ml (1 pint) heat-treated milk (see above)
1 tablespoon freshly bought natural yoghurt

method

1 Heat the milk to 43°C (109°F) or until you can dip a clean finger in it for just 10 seconds. Add the yoghurt and mix well.

2 Pour into a clean, pre-warmed vacuum flask or into the containers of an electric yoghurt-maker. Close and leave undisturbed for 8–10 hours to allow the yoghurt to set.

3 Store in the fridge and use as required.

 makes 600ml (1 pint)

porridge

On a cold winter's morning, nothing is more warming than a steaming bowl of porridge. The Scots traditionally use oats but you can make interesting porridge with a variety of different cereals.

oat porridge

Rolled or porridge oats make the quickest porridge. This is usually ready in 3–5 minutes, depending on the size of the flakes. You can also use oatmeal but it takes longer to cook.

ingredients
250–275ml (9–9½fl oz) skimmed milk, soya or rice milk
250–275ml (9–9½fl oz) water
75g (3oz) porridge oats
2 teaspoons honey
1 tablespoon mixed flax (linseed) and pumpkin seeds, freshly ground

method **1** Pour the milk and the water into a saucepan and sprinkle in the oats. Bring to the boil and simmer for 4–5 minutes, stirring all the time.

2 Serve with the honey and the ground seed mixture.

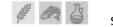 serves 2

millet or rice flake porridge

Both these flaked cereals cook as quickly, if not faster, than porridge oats. The resulting porridges tend to be smoother (more like semolina) and without such a definite flavour, so flavourings are important.

ingredients 75g (3oz) flaked rice or millet
400–450ml (14–16fl oz) half-and-half skimmed milk or soya milk and water
nutmeg or vanilla essence (to taste)
2 teaspoons honey
1 tablespoon five-seed mix (see page 43), freshly ground

method **1** Cook in just the same way as the Oat Porridge, adding the nutmeg or vanilla flavouring at the beginning of the cooking time.

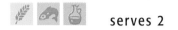 serves 2

quinoa porridge with bananas

If you haven't tried quinoa yet, you should. It is extremely versatile and nutritious. Here it is in its breakfast guise.

ingredients 75g (3oz) quinoa
freshly grated nutmeg
2–3 tablespoons soya or rice milk
4 tablespoons low-fat natural live yoghurt
1 banana, peeled and sliced

method **1** Place the quinoa in a saucepan with 350–375ml (12–13fl oz) water and bring to the boil. Cover and simmer for 15 minutes. The mixture should still be quite sloppy.

2 Tip the mixture into a blender and process with the nutmeg and soya or rice milk. Add more liquid if needed to give a porridge-like consistency.

3 Return the mixture to the pan and gently reheat. Serve topped with a couple of spoonfuls of yoghurt and some sliced banana.

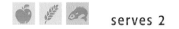 serves 2

eggs

healthy scrambled eggs

While eggs are rather high in fat, they are also a good source of protein and can add variety to your diet. Serve them occasionally as part of a more substantial breakfast.

ingredients

2 large free-range eggs
2 tablespoons skimmed or soya milk
2 tablespoons freshly chopped parsley

a knob of butter
2 slices whole rye toast

method

1 Beat the eggs with the milk and parsley.

2 Melt the butter in a small saucepan. Pour in the egg mixture and cook slowly over a low heat, stirring constantly. Serve on whole rye toast.

 serves 2

breakfast omelettes

This omelette is a very quick way of serving eggs. Fillings add extra nutrients, as well as interest.

ingredients

3 free-range eggs
3 tablespoons skimmed or soya milk
a knob of butter
a filling (e.g. 2 tablespoons mixed beansprouts, 1 finely chopped tomato, ½ finely chopped red pepper, 2 tablespoons canned sweetcorn or Mexicorn)

method

1 Beat the eggs and milk in a bowl. Heat the butter in a small non-stick frying pan and pour in the egg mixture. Carefully stir the egg to fold the mixture a little.

2 When it is nearly set, sprinkle on your chosen filling and fold over. Cut in half to serve.

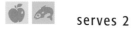 serves 2

light meals

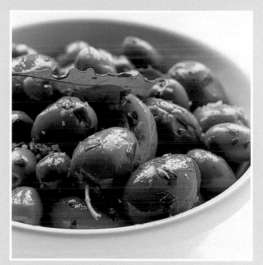

cold light meals

winter salad platter with tangy cucumber dressing

Most root vegetables are delicious if they are simply grated and eaten raw. This way you also receive their full vitamin content. For a change, try celeriac, turnip, kholrabi or white radish in place of one of the vegetables used here.

The lightly toasted nuts and seeds add flavour and a crunchy texture but take care not to burn them.

ingredients

TANGY CUCUMBER DRESSING
7–10cm (3–4in) length of cucumber, chopped
25g (1oz) low-fat natural live yoghurt
2 spring onions, roughly chopped
½ clove garlic, peeled and chopped
2 teaspoons cider vinegar
½ teaspoon Dijon mustard
a few drops Worcester sauce
2 teaspoons freshly chopped dill
½ teaspoon celery seeds (optional)

WINTER SALAD PLATTER
2 heads chicory, trimmed and sliced
100g (3½oz) cabbage greens or sprout tops, very finely shredded
200g (7oz) carrots, peeled and finely grated
1 teaspoon lemon juice
2 medium-sized uncooked beetroot, peeled and finely grated
200g (7oz) uncooked parsnip, peeled and finely grated
2 tablespoons mixed lightly toasted sunflower seeds and flaked almonds or
    pine nuts

method   **1** Start by making the Cucumber Dressing. Place all the ingredients in a blender and process until smooth. If possible, refrigerate for an hour or so (in order to blend the flavours). Whisk lightly with a fork before using.

2 Mix the sliced chicory and cabbage greens together and arrange on two serving plates.

3 Mix the carrot with a little lemon juice to prevent it from discoloring.

4 Arrange small mounds of the carrot and grated vegetables on top of the cabbage greens and chicory. Then pour on the Cucumber Dressing, sprinkle with the toasted seeds and nuts and serve at once.

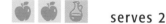 serves 2

brussels sprouts and nut salad

This wonderfully crunchy, detoxifying salad makes a good light lunch. Follow it with fresh fruit or dates stuffed with low-fat soft cheese.

ingredients
    150g (5½ oz) Brussels sprouts, trimmed and thinly sliced
    12 radishes, trimmed and sliced
    3cm (1½ in) length of cucumber, diced
    50g (2oz) lightly toasted almonds or cashews
    2 tablespoons freshly chopped parsley
    2 tablespoons cold-pressed mixed seed oil
    2 tablespoons lemon juice

method   **1** Prepare the vegetables and mix together in a bowl. Divide the mixture between two serving bowls and top with the toasted nuts and parsley.

2 Mix the seed oil and lemon juice together, pour over the top of the salad mix and serve.

 serves 2

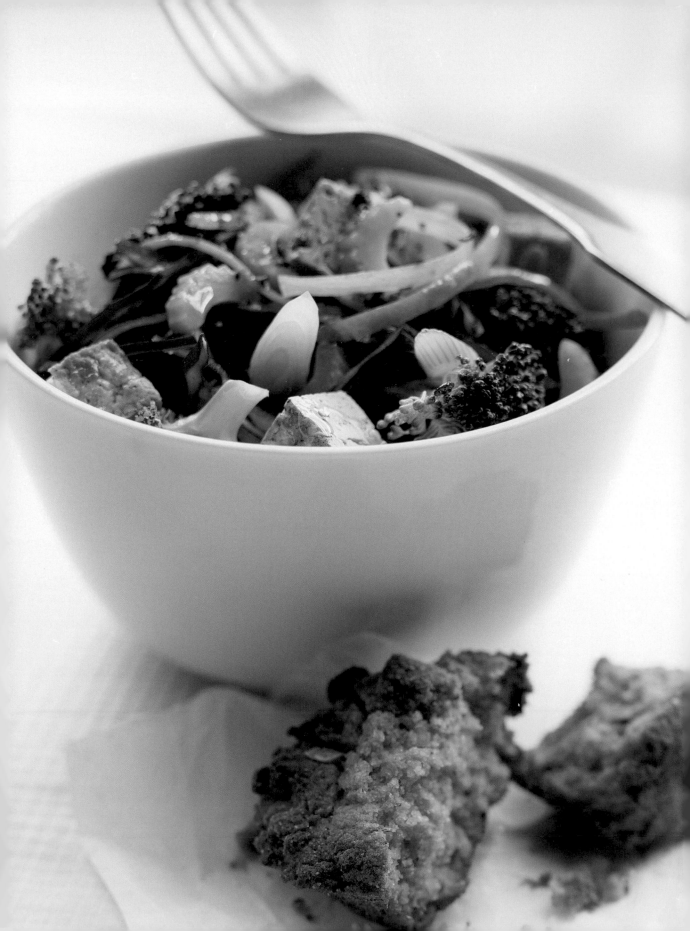

red cabbage and mixed vegetable salad
with tofu

You can make this colourful, crunchy salad at any time of the year. Serve it with Rye Bread or home-made Herby Corn Bread (see page 48).

Ingredients

75g (3oz) red cabbage, chopped
75g (3oz) broccoli florets, chopped
2 medium carrots, scrubbed and grated
2 sticks celery, sliced
2 spring onions, chopped
150g (5½oz) smoked or marinated tofu, diced

DRESSING
2 tablespoons cold-pressed mixed seed oil
1 tablespoon lemon juice or cider vinegar
freshly ground black pepper (to taste)

method

1 Combine all the salad ingredients in a large bowl.

2 Mix the dressing ingredients of the salad together and pour over the top separately. Toss together and serve at once.

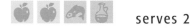 serves 2

chicken salad with horseradish sauce

The horseradish sauce in this filling, main-course salad recipe is both piquant and refreshing. It would also make a good dressing for much simpler side salads, to serve with roasts or grills.

ingredients

2 Little Gem lettuces, shredded
200–250g (7–9oz) cooked chicken meat without the skin, cut into chunks
2 medium potatoes, steamed in their skins, peeled, cooled and sliced
1 eating apple, cubed
5cm (2in) length of cucumber, sliced
8 cherry tomatoes, halved
a few sprigs of fresh parsley or dill
paprika pepper (to taste)

HORSERADISH SAUCE
3 heaped tablespoons low-fat natural live yoghurt
1 tablespoon horseradish sauce
3 tablespoons lemon juice
3 tablespoons skimmed milk or water

method

1 Place the shredded lettuce on two serving plates. Arrange the chicken, sliced potatoes, apple, cucumber and tomatoes on top of the lettuce.

2 Mix all the Horseradish Sauce ingredients in a cup and spoon over the salads. Decorate with the fresh herbs and a sprinkling of paprika pepper.

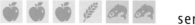 serves 2

beansprout and chicory salad
with roquefort

I like to serve this attractive salad with rye crispbread. If you are feeling particularly hungry, finish the meal with a slice of Lexia Raisin Flapjack (see page 94).

ingredients

1 head chicory, broken into spears
100g (3½ oz) mixed beansprouts
40g (1½ oz) walnuts, broken into pieces
75g (3oz) Roquefort cheese, crumbled

DRESSING
2 tablespoons cold-pressed mixed seed oil
1 tablespoon extra-virgin olive oil
2 teaspoons raspberry vinegar
Solo salt and freshly ground black pepper (to taste)

method

1 Arrange the chicory spears in circles on two serving plates and top with a mound of mixed beansprouts. Sprinkle with the walnuts and cheese.

2 Put all the dressing ingredients in a small jug and beat well with a fork. Just before serving, pour the dressing over the salad.

 serves 2

beetroot and smoked herring salad with spinach and fennel salad

English oak-smoked herrings are widely available but you might also come across German juniper-smoked herrings in some shops. These give a more exotic, slightly aniseed flavour to the salad.

ingredients

BEETROOT AND SMOKED HERRING SALAD
1 small smoked herring
1 large cooked beetroot, peeled and diced
1 sweet sour pickled cucumber, diced
1 small apple, cored and diced
3 tablespoons low-fat natural live yoghurt

SPINACH AND FENNEL SALAD
125g (4oz) baby spinach leaves
1 medium courgette, thinly sliced
¼ head of fennel, sliced and very finely chopped

DRESSING
1 tablespoon extra-virgin olive oil
1 teaspoon cider vinegar
2 sun-dried tomatoes, cut into thin strips

method

1 To make the Beetroot and Smoked Herring Salad, skin the herring and remove the flesh from the bones. Flake and add to the vegetables and apple. Mix together with the yoghurt and pile onto two serving plates.

2 For the Spinach and Fennel Salad, place all the salad ingredients in a bowl. Mix all the dressing ingredients in a cup and spoon over the salad.

3 Toss well and serve on the side with the Beetroot and Smoked Herring Salad.

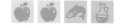

serves 2

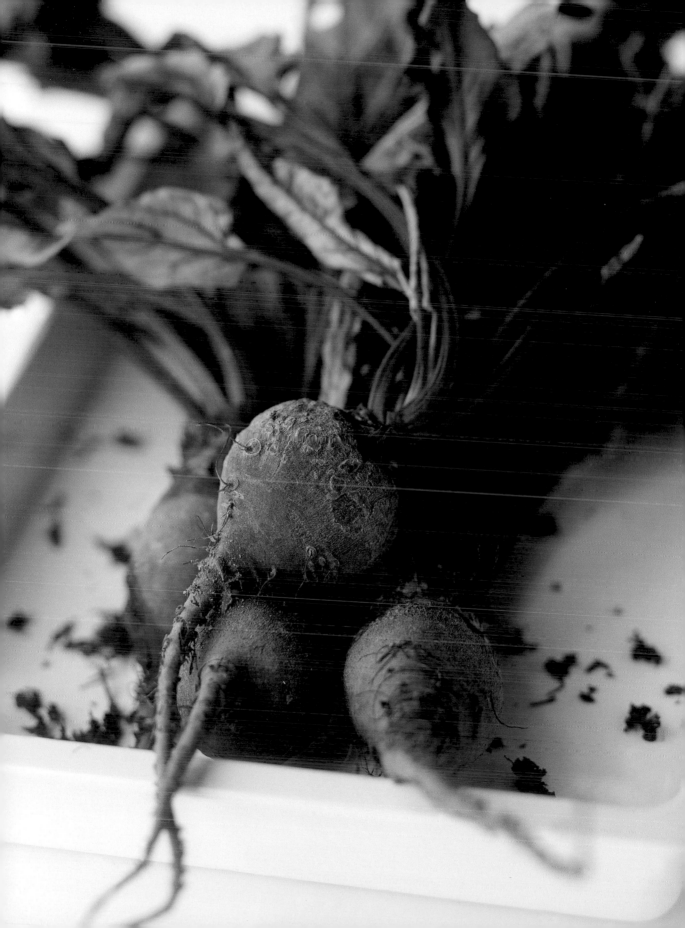

hot light meals

steam-fry vegetables with green curry paste

Don't worry if you don't have all the ingredients listed for this very versatile dish – simply substitute the vegetables that you do have to hand. Cauliflower, beans, broccoli, sugar snap peas, mangetout and asparagus can all be used.

We have used a proprietary Thai green curry paste for this recipe. You can, of course, make up your own Thai mix of spices but it is quite expensive to buy all the ingredients and, unless you regularly make Thai dishes, they can go to waste. Look out for brands which do not use any additives – check the ingredients list.

The basics of steam-frying are set out on page 34. This method ensures the lightest of cooking with the minimum of fat.

ingredients

1 onion, peeled and sliced

2 cloves garlic, peeled and chopped

1 teaspoon extra-virgin olive oil

2–3 tablespoons water or vegetable stock

2–3 tablespoons green curry paste (to taste)

1 red pepper, seeded and cut into strips

6–8 baby courgettes, cut in half lengthways, *or* 1 large courgette, cut into sticks

6–8 patty pan courgettes, trimmed and cut in half

300g (10½ oz) tofu, cubed

1 carrot, shaved with a large potato peeler

100g (3½ oz) brown cap or shiitake mushrooms, sliced

2 tablespoons coconut milk

150g (5½ oz) beansprouts

fresh coriander (to garnish)

method

1 Quickly steam-fry the onion and garlic in the oil and then in the water or stock for 2–3 minutes. Stir in the green curry paste and add the pepper, courgettes and patty pan courgettes. Continue to steam-fry for another 3–4 minutes.

2 Add all the remaining ingredients, except the beansprouts and coriander, and toss carefully in the pan juices. Cook until the vegetables are cooked but still firm to the bite.

3 Stir in the beansprouts, toss and serve with rice or noodles. Garnish with sprigs of fresh coriander.

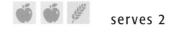 **serves 2**

brunch rosti

You can buy packs of ready-made Swiss rosti but they tend to have a rather metallic flavour and may contain preservatives. Alternatively, you can make Swiss rosti from scratch but this involves a good deal of preparation, with an overnight standing period.

This recipe for Brunch Rosti is much quicker and easier, but it does include egg and so may not be suitable for everyone. Serve it with grilled mushrooms and tomatoes.

ingredients

2 potatoes, peeled
1 onion, peeled and very finely chopped
1 large (size 1) egg, beaten
1 dessertspoon plain flour
a little extra-virgin olive oil

method

1 Grate the potatoes into a bowl and quickly mix with the onion, egg and flour. Heat a heavy-based pan and brush with the oil. Drop four spoonfuls of the rosti mixture into the hot pan.

2 Reduce the heat and cook for about 10–12 minutes until the base of the rosti is golden. Turn over and cook on the other side until it too is golden in colour. Serve immediately.

serves 2

feta stuffed mushrooms

Tofu can be used here in place of the Feta cheese but you will need to add some soy sauce and perhaps a little freshly grated ginger to the stuffing mixture to achieve a similarly punchy flavour.

Serve with Brunch Rosti (see page 63) or with Stuffed Tomatoes (see page 124) if you cannot eat eggs.

ingredients

4 field mushrooms or large open-cap mushrooms
150ml (5fl oz) half-and-half white wine and water
75g (3oz) Feta cheese, mashed with a fork
2 tablespoons sesame seeds
2 tablespoons freshly chopped parsley
2 tablespoons dry breadcrumbs
freshly ground black pepper (to taste)
a few sprigs of fresh parsley

method

1 Place the mushrooms in a shallow pan and pour in the wine and water. Bring the mixture to the boil and cover with a lid. Cook for about 15 minutes until the mushrooms have softened and most of the liquid has been absorbed.

2 Place the mushrooms on a large piece of foil. Mix any remaining cooking liquor with the Feta cheese, sesame seeds, parsley, breadcrumbs and pepper. Spoon the mixture over the gills of the mushrooms and place under a hot grill.

3 Cook for 3–4 minutes until the cheese is lightly browned and serve at once on a bed of rosti, garnished with sprigs of fresh parsley.

 serves 2

spanish rice with fennel

This is such a quick and easy recipe to make that when I am working at home I have it regularly. It's good served with watercress or a green salad on the side.

ingredients

75–100g (3–3½oz) rice
1 x 400g (14oz) can tomatoes
2 small onions, peeled and sliced into rounds
1 small red pepper, seeded and sliced
2 small heads fennel, trimmed and sliced
freshly ground black pepper (to taste)

method

1 Place the rice in a 15cm (7in) shallow pan. Pour the tomatoes and their juice over the top. Then arrange the onion and pepper rings with the fennel on top of the tomatoes and sprinkle with black pepper.

2 Bring to the boil and when the mixture is bubbling well, reduce the heat. Cover with a well-fitting lid and leave to cook for about 20–25 minutes until the rice is tender and has absorbed almost all the liquid. Brown rice may take a little longer. Serve from the pan.

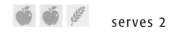

serves 2

devilled tomatoes on polenta squares

Here's an answer for those people who would like to make quick 'on toast' snacks but are allergic to wheat. Cold-cooked polenta slices make an excellent substitute for bread – you can buy the mixture in large squares or sausage shapes ready to slice.

ingredients

2 large or 4 small slices cooked polenta

6 tomatoes, cut in half horizontally

2 tablespoons extra-virgin olive oil, plus extra for brushing

1 clove garlic, peeled and crushed

½ teaspoon dry mustard powder

¼ teaspoon cumin powder

¼ teaspoon curry powder

2 tablespoons mango chutney

method

1 Brush the polenta slices with oil and grill them on each side for 5–6 minutes.

2 Place the tomato halves on a large piece of foil, cut side down, and place under a hot grill for 3–4 minutes until the skins just begin to char.

3 Turn the tomatoes over. Mix 2 tablespoons oil with the garlic, mustard powder and spices and spoon a little of the mixture over each cut surface of tomato. Return to the grill for another 3–4 minutes.

4 Spread some mango chutney on each slice of polenta, top with the curried tomato mixture, and serve.

 serves 2

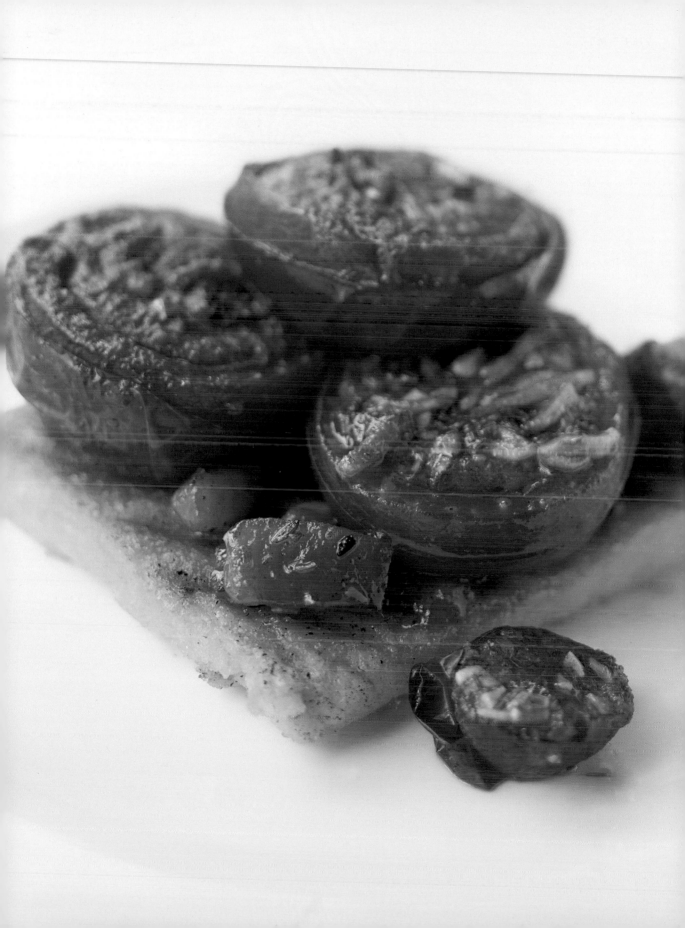

lemon chicken on leafy asparagus salad

If you like, you can use firm fish fillets such as tuna or salmon or fried tofu, in place of the chicken in this lovely warm recipe. Serve with good crusty rolls or Tomato Scofa Bread (see page 46).

ingredients

1 large chicken breast, skinned and boned
juice of ½ lemon
1 clove garlic, peeled and crushed
1 stick lemon grass *or* 1 teaspoon dried chopped lemon grass
freshly ground black pepper (to taste)
1 teaspoon cold-pressed mixed seed oil
100g (3½ oz) asparagus spears
8 baby courgettes
100g (3½ oz) mixed salad leaves
1 tablespoon lightly toasted flaked almonds or pine nuts

method

1 Cut the chicken into thin strips, put it into a non-metallic bowl and mix it with the lemon juice, garlic, lemon grass, black pepper and cold-pressed mixed seed oil. Cover and refrigerate until required.

2 Place the asparagus and courgettes in the top of a steamer over boiling water and cook for about 5 minutes to soften slightly.

3 Arrange the mixed leaves on two serving plates and top with the lightly cooked vegetables.

4 Brush a non-stick wok with a little more oil and steam-fry the chicken pieces, using the strained marinade to moisten the pan after a minute or two.

5 Cover with a lid and leave on the heat for about 8 minutes until the chicken is cooked through.

6 Spoon the chicken and the pan juices over the salad. Sprinkle with the nuts and serve at once.

 serves 2

oriental vegetables with tofu

You can buy red fermented bean curd in tins at most Chinese grocers. Failing that, you can use miso paste or instant miso soup mix. It goes without saying that the latter will not taste quite the same!

ingredients

1 small cube of red fermented bean curd
1 ½ tablespoons olive oil
150g (5½ oz) canned bamboo shoots
150g (5½ oz) canned lotus roots, cut into 0.5cm (¼ in) slices
1 large clove garlic, peeled and finely chopped
150g (5½ oz) mushrooms, sliced
1 teaspoon soy sauce
1 teaspoon sesame oil
1 teaspoon vegetable stock
3 pieces deep-fried tofu slices, approximately 300g (10½ oz)
2 spring onions, trimmed and sliced
a few sprigs of fresh coriander (to garnish)

method

1 Mix the red fermented bean curd with 50ml (2fl oz) water and 1 teaspoon of the olive oil. Bring the mixture to the boil and add the bamboo shoots and lotus roots. Stir and cook slowly for 3 minutes. Cover and keep warm.

2 Heat the remaining oil in a saucepan and stir-fry the garlic for a few seconds. Add the mushrooms and continue to stir-fry for 2–3 minutes. Add the soy sauce and ½ teaspoon sesame oil. Reduce the heat and cook for another 2 minutes. Keep warm on one side.

3 Put 50ml (2fl oz) water in a pan with the vegetable stock and bring to the boil. Add the rest of the sesame oil and the tofu slices. Cook for 2 minutes.

4 To serve, arrange the tofu in the centre of a large dish and surround with the bamboo shoots and lotus roots. Pour the mushrooms and their juices over the top. Garnish with the spring onions and coriander.

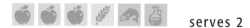

serves 2

smoked haddock kedgeree with grilled tomatoes

The tomatoes give this traditional brunch recipe a moist texture. If you prefer a softer kedgeree you could stir in some Greek yoghurt or silken tofu. Vegans can easily substitute smoked tofu for smoked haddock.

ingredients

150g (5½ oz) undyed smoked haddock fillet
1 egg
100g (3½ oz) brown basmati rice
2 large Continental tomatoes
1 clove of garlic, crushed (optional)
2 tablespoons freshly chopped parsley
paprika pepper (to taste)

method

1 Place the fish in a small pan with about 50ml (2fl oz) water. Cover with a lid and steam for about 7–8 minutes, depending on the thickness of the fillet. Hard-boil the egg, then peel and chop it.

2 Place 250ml (9fl oz) water in a pan and bring to the boil. Add the rice, stir and cover with a lid. Reduce the heat and leave to cook for about 20–25 minutes, when the rice should be cooked and all the water absorbed.

3 Meanwhile, cut the tomatoes in half and sprinkle with the garlic, if using, pushing it into the watery, seedy area to stop it burning. Place under a hot grill and cook for 5–6 minutes.

4 Fluff up the rice with a fork and stir in the cooked haddock, hard-boiled egg and parsley. Sprinkle with the paprika and serve with the grilled tomatoes.

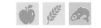 **serves 2**

provençal vegetables with goat's cheese dressing

This dish from Ursula Ferrigno, author of Real Fast Food, *captures the flavour of Provence. She likes to serve the vegetables when they are still just warm so that the flavour of the dressing is absorbed.*

ingredients

75g (3oz) French beans
8 baby courgettes
75g (3oz) mangetout
75g (3oz) broccoli florets
a handful of lightly toasted pine nuts

DRESSING
2–3 ripe tomatoes, peeled and roughly chopped
40g (1 ½ oz) soft mild goat's cheese
½ clove garlic, peeled and chopped
2 tablespoons extra-virgin olive oil
½ tablespoon lemon juice
a little salt and pepper (to taste)

method

1 Start by making the dressing. Put the tomatoes in a blender with the goat's cheese, garlic, olive oil, lemon juice and seasonings. Process until smooth.

2 In a large saucepan of boiling water, blanch the vegetables in batches until just tender but firm to the bite. Remove from the pan with a slotted spoon and drain very well on kitchen paper.

3 To serve, put the vegetables in a bowl, pour over the dressing and garnish with the toasted pine nuts.

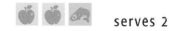 serves 2

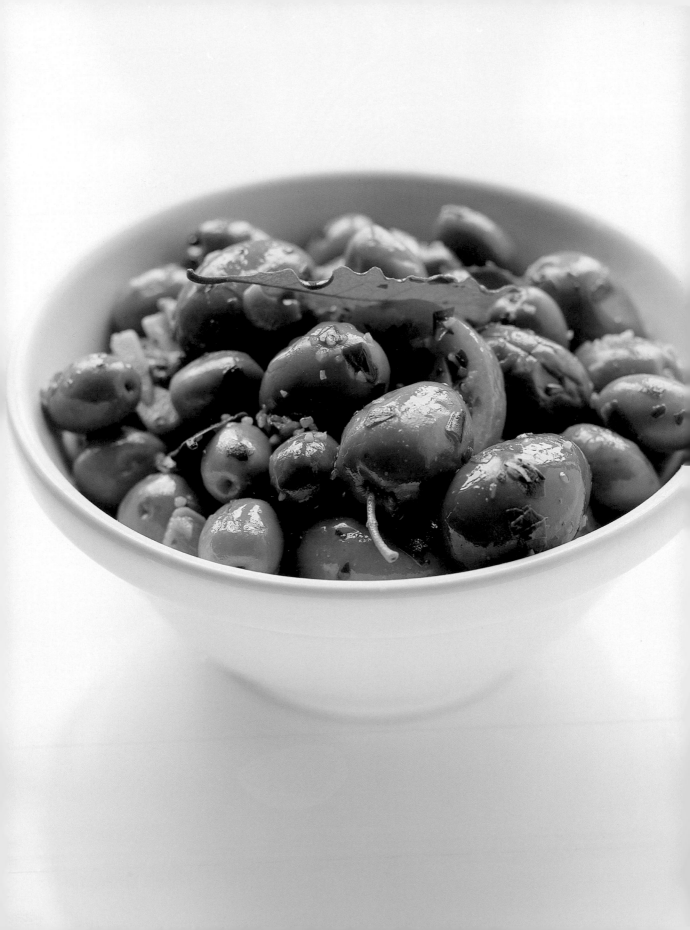

spaghetti pomodoro with olives

Typical of southern Italy, this dish is healthy, quick and colourful. You can use fresh tomatoes in summer but substitute canned tomatoes in winter when we do not have the lovely ripe tomatoes which are available in Puglia for most of the year.

This recipe makes about 300ml (10fl oz) sauce so you might able to keep some for another day. It's certainly a useful standby whenever Tomato Sauce is required. It also freezes very well.

ingredients

1 large onion, peeled and chopped

1 clove of garlic, peeled and crushed

700g (1½lb) fresh tomatoes, skinned and sliced, *or* 2 x 400g (14oz) cans tomatoes

2 tablespoons tomato purée

salt and freshly ground black pepper (to taste)

2 teaspoons freshly chopped basil

spaghetti (to serve 2)

16–20 small black olives

method

1 Put the onion and garlic in a saucepan and barely cover with water. Bring to the boil and simmer for about five to seven minutes until soft. Add the tomatoes, tomato purée and seasoning and return to the boil.

2 Lower the heat and simmer for 35–40 minutes in a partially covered pan so that the sauce reduces, but keep an eye on it to make sure that it does not burn. Stir in the basil. Use the sauce as it is, or purée if you prefer a smoother texture.

3 Cook the pasta as directed on the pack and drain well. Toss with the olives, spoon the tomato sauce over the top and serve.

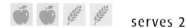 serves 2

quinoa pilaf with chickpeas and dried fruits

This recipe is also very good made with bulgar wheat in place of quinoa. You may also like to try it with whole millet. If you do use these other grains you may need to adjust the amount of liquid.

ingredients

1 teaspoon extra-virgin olive oil
1 medium onion, peeled and coarsely chopped
2 small sticks celery, trimmed and chopped
2 small leeks, trimmed and chopped
125g (4oz) canned chickpeas (drained weight)
1 stick of cinnamon
4 cardamom pods
100g (3½oz) quinoa
250ml (9fl oz) vegetable stock or water
25g (1oz) sunflower seeds
25g (1oz) raisins
6 prunes
grated zest of ½ lemon
some freshly chopped parsley

method

1 Brush the base of a deep non-stick frying pan with the oil. Add the onion, celery and leeks to the pan and cook gently for about 3 minutes to release the flavours. Keep the vegetables on the move with a wooden spoon and do not allow them to brown.

2 Add the chickpeas, spices, quinoa and vegetable stock or water to the mixture in the pan and stir. Bring to the boil, cover the pan and cook over a low heat for 10 minutes.

3 Add the sunflower seeds, raisins, prunes and lemon zest, and continue cooking for another 10 minutes until all the liquid has been absorbed and the quinoa is cooked through.

4 Pile the pilaf onto two serving plates, tossing gently to separate the grains. Sprinkle with plenty of freshly chopped parsley and serve at once.

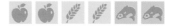

serves 2

hot and spicy pepper chicken with green herb salad

Serve this versatile dish with freshly cooked brown rice.

ingredients

1 medium onion, peeled and roughly chopped
1 clove garlic, peeled and crushed
1 small green chilli pepper, seeded and finely chopped
2 chicken breasts, skinned and boned
1 green pepper, seeded and chopped
1 red pepper, seeded and chopped
1 tablespoon Cajun spicy sauce, Harissa, Thai red curry paste or Szechuan stir-fry sauce (to taste)
freshly ground black pepper (to taste)
25g (1oz) mangetout

GREEN HERB SALAD

50g (2oz) rocket
50g (2oz) corn lettuce
25g (1oz) broadleaf parsley
15g (½oz) fresh mint
juice of ½ lemon
a little cold-preserved mixed seed oil (optional)

method

1 Steam-fry (see page 34) the onion, garlic and green chilli in a non-stick frying pan.

2 Cut the chicken into fairly thin strips and add to the pan with the onion mixture. Cook for another 5 minutes, stirring continually.

3 Now add the peppers and spicy sauce. Toss everything together, season and cover with a lid. Cook for another 10 minutes. Add the mangetout for the last 3 minutes of the cooking time.

4 Make the Green Herb Salad just before serving. Simply toss the salad leaves and herbs together and pile into two salad bowls. Sprinkle the salad with the lemon juice or with a mixture of lemon juice and mixed seed oil. Serve at once with the Hot and Spicy Chicken.

serves 2

warm mackerel salad with avocado and mango served with honey-toasted sunflower seeds

There are plenty of essential fatty acids in this wonderfully colourful salad from Carlton Food Network chef Peter Vaughan, and the honey-toasted sunflower seeds are a real treat.

ingredients

4 small fillets cooked smoked mackerel
1 ripe mango, pitted, peeled and sliced
1 ripe avocado pear, pitted, peeled and sliced
assorted salad leaves
1 dessertspoon cold-pressed sunflower oil
50g (2oz) sunflower seeds
2 teaspoons runny honey

DRESSING
1 tablespoon extra-virgin olive oil
juice of ½ lemon
2 teaspoons Dijon mustard
1 teaspoon creamed horseradish relish
a bunch of fresh chives, chopped

method

1 Using a sharp knife, cut the middle part of each mackerel fillet either side of the pin bones. This will help you to remove any remaining bones in the fish. Place the fillets under the grill for six to seven minutes to heat through.

2 Mix the mango, avocado and salad leaves together. Then mix all the dressing ingredients in a bowl with a wire whisk and use to dress the salad. Arrange on two serving plates.

3 Heat the sunflower oil in a small frying pan. When it is really hot and just about to smoke, add the sunflower seeds and let them toast for a minute or two. When the seeds have turned golden, quickly add the honey and remove from the heat.

4 Place the warm mackerel fillets on the prepared salad and top with the honey-toasted sunflower seeds.

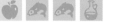 **serves 2**

snacks

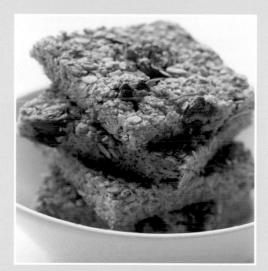

sandwiches

flaked salmon and dill open sandwiches
on rye

Don't waste time trying to pick out the skin and bones from the canned salmon. This is where much of the calcium is, so eat the lot!

ingredients

2 x 213g (7½oz) can red salmon, drained
2 tablespoons freshly chopped dill
2 tablespoons low-fat natural live yoghurt
freshly ground black pepper (to taste)
2 large slices rye bread
1 large or 2 small pickled cucumbers, sliced
4 radishes, sliced
a few sprigs of watercress

method

1 Mash the salmon in a bowl and mix in the dill, yoghurt and pepper.

2 Pile the mixture onto the rye bread and decorate with alternate slices of pickled cucumber and radish and sprigs of watercress.

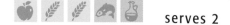

serves 2

cottage cheese open sandwiches with
watercress and sesame seeds

Good open sandwiches have colour and texture as well as healthy ingredients so take care when arranging the sprigs of watercress on the cheese and sesame base. And make sure you don't burn the seeds when toasting them – they should just be a light golden colour.

ingredients
2 thick slices wholemeal bread
150g (5½oz) cottage cheese
2 tablespoons lightly toasted sesame seeds
50g (2oz) watercress
6 radishes, sliced

method **1** Cut each slice of bread in half, spread with the cottage cheese and sprinkle with sesame seeds. Arrange the sprigs of watercress on top, pressing them into the cheese. Dot with the sliced radishes and serve.

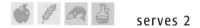 serves 2

hummus, cucumber and alfalfa sprouts
on rye crispbread

Eat these crispbread open sandwiches as soon as they are made. If you leave them to stand they will soon lose their crispness.

ingredients
150g (5½oz) hummus
4 rye crispbreads
1 small whole cucumber, sliced
alfalfa sprouts (to taste)
8 black olives

method **1** Spread the hummus thickly and evenly over each slice of crispbread. Arrange slices of cucumber on the hummus and heap the alfalfa sprouts on top. Decorate with the black olives and serve.

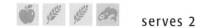 serves 2

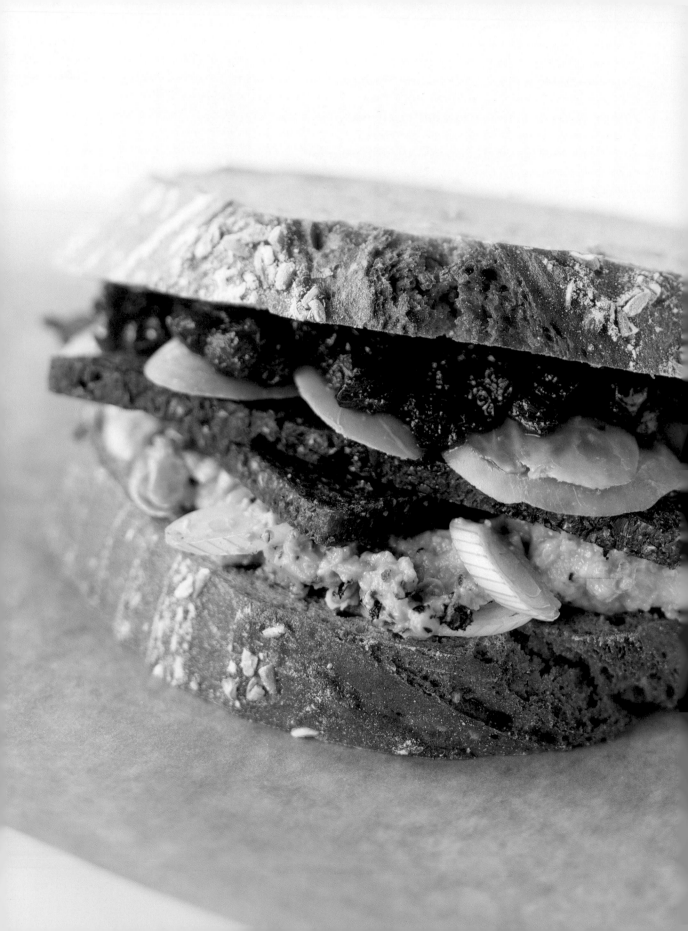

rye deckers with avocado, smoked chicken and cranberry sauce

This combination of ingredients may sound a little unusual but they work wonderfully together. The secret is to choose a really ripe avocado and a cranberry sauce which is not too sweet.

ingredients

1 ripe avocado, peeled and pitted

2 teaspoons lemon juice

2–3 spring onions, trimmed and very finely chopped

ground black pepper (to taste)

a little butter or non-hydrogenated vegetable margarine

4 slices rye bread

2 slices pumpernickel

1–1½ tablespoons cranberry sauce

1 smoked chicken leg joint, skinned and sliced

method

1 Mash the avocado with the lemon juice and mix in the spring onions and black pepper.

2 Very lightly butter all the pieces of bread and cut them to the same size. Place two slices of rye bread on a board or work surface and spread with the avocado mixture.

3 Spread each slice of pumpernickel with the cranberry sauce and place on top of the avocado. Arrange the sliced chicken on the cranberry sauce and top with the remaining slices of rye bread. Cut in half to serve.

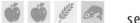 serves 2

provençal tuna salad in a bun

Known as Pain Bagnat *in the South of France, these buns are more of a meal than a snack!*

ingredients

2 large sesame buns, split in half

1–2 tablespoons extra-virgin olive oil

8–10 soft lettuce leaves

1 good-sized Continental tomato or 2 ordinary tomatoes, sliced

1 x 100g (3½ oz) can of tuna in olive oil, drained and flaked

1 very small onion, peeled and thinly sliced

½ small red pepper, seeded and cut into rings

12 black olives (optional)

method

1 Brush each half of the bun with olive oil. Place the bases on a board and arrange the lettuce leaves and tomato slices on them. Next, add the tuna and onion and pepper rings.

2 Add more olive oil to taste and dot with black olives, if using. Place the second half of the bun on top and press down well. Serve at once. Warn everyone about the olive stones!

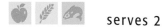

serves 2

beetroot and tahini special

This combination makes very good open or closed sandwiches. Simply add some more sprigs of mint and a slice of cucumber to decorate the open variety. Choose any bread that suits your dietary requirements.

ingredients

50g (2oz) watercress, chopped

3–4 good sprigs of fresh mint, chopped

2 level tablespoons tahini paste

lemon juice (to taste)

2–4 slices bread

1 medium cooked beetroot, sliced

method **1** Mix the chopped watercress and mint with the tahini paste in a basin and add a little lemon juice to taste.

2 Spread the mixture over two of the slices of bread and top with the sliced beetroot.

3 Decorate with mint and cucumber or cover with another slice of bread to make a closed sandwich.

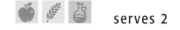 serves 2

danish herrings on rye with gherkins and beetroot

There is a very wide range of Scandinavian pickled herrings available these days. Choose sweet-pickled or mustard-pickled herrings or onion-stuffed rollmops for a change.

ingredients
2 large slices rye bread or pumpernickel
a little butter
1 large cooked beetroot, sliced
150g (5½ oz) Danish curried herrings
4 cocktail gherkins, cut into fan shapes
4 sprigs of fresh dill

method **1** Spread the slices of rye bread or pumpernickel sparingly with butter and cut each in half.

2 Arrange the beetroot slices at one end of each slice and the pieces of curried herring at the other. Decorate with the gherkin fans and sprigs of dill, and serve.

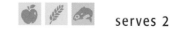 serves 2

dips

You may think that dips are too much trouble to make for a quick snack, but if you use a blender you can rustle them up in minutes. They make a really healthy snack served with raw vegetable crudités or perhaps organic nachos for a change.

spicy red bean dip

I like this spicy red bean dip to have a slightly lumpy texture but, if you prefer, you can add a little more yoghurt and blend until smooth and creamy. Serve with a selection of carrot and parsnip sticks.

ingredients
150g (5½oz) canned red kidney beans, rinsed and drained
75g (3oz) cottage cheese
3 small spring onions, trimmed and chopped
1 clove garlic, peeled and chopped
1 tablespoon low-fat natural live yoghurt
1 teaspoon extra-virgin olive oil
a pinch of chilli powder or a few drops of Tabasco

method **1** Place all the ingredients in a blender and process until you get the required texture.

serves 2

avocado and tofu dip

If you use silken tofu you may not need quite as much soya milk to get the desired creaminess. Carrot sticks go particularly well with the flavours of this dip but you can use any fresh vegetables that come to hand. Prepare the crudités last.

ingredients   150g (5½ oz) silken or ordinary tofu
1 small ripe avocado
1 large clove garlic, peeled and crushed
2–3 spring onions, trimmed and finely chopped
2 tablespoons freshly chopped parsley
1 teaspoon tamari or soy sauce
freshly ground black pepper (to taste)
75–150ml (3–5fl oz) soya milk

method   **1** Process all the ingredients in a blender until smooth, adding as much soya milk as you need to achieve the desired consistency.

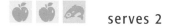 serves 2

smoked mackerel dip

Rich in Omega 3 oils, smoked mackerel should find a ready place in your diet. Use it in sandwich toppings, in salads or in this creamy dip accompanied by celery, carrot and cucumber sticks.

ingredients   100g (3½ oz) smoked mackerel fillet
150g (5½ oz) thick yoghurt
2 tablespoons lemon juice
a little grated lemon rind
plenty of black pepper

method   **1** Place all the ingredients in a blender, whizz until smooth and serve.

 serves 2

sprouting beans and seeds

The best way to sprout beans and seeds at home is to buy a layered bean-sprouter which allows you to pour water in at the top and catch the drips at the base. However, it is also possible to use a jam jar or, for larger quantities, a kilner jar.

- Soak your chosen beans or seeds in cold water for 12 hours or overnight. Take care to use only 1–2 dessertspoons beans or seeds for they will soon swell and grow to fill the space in your sprouter.

- The next day, drain the beans or seeds and place in your sprouter. If you are using a jar, close it with a perforated lid or with a double layer of muslin held in place by a rubber band. Place on a sloping draining board so that any excess liquid can drain out.

- Water your sprouting beans or seeds twice a day and allow them to drain in between. The sprouts will be ready in three or four days.

What to Sprout?

Adzuki Beans
Use particularly small quantities as these beans really increase in volume. Harvest after four or five days.

Alfalfa Seeds
These require only six hours' soaking time and grow into a fine, cress-like vegetable. Harvest after three to six days.

Barley
Difficult to sprout at home and usually best served cooked. Harvest after three or four days when the sprout is still quite small.

Black-eyed Beans
These provide crisp and juicy sprouts. Harvest after three to five days.

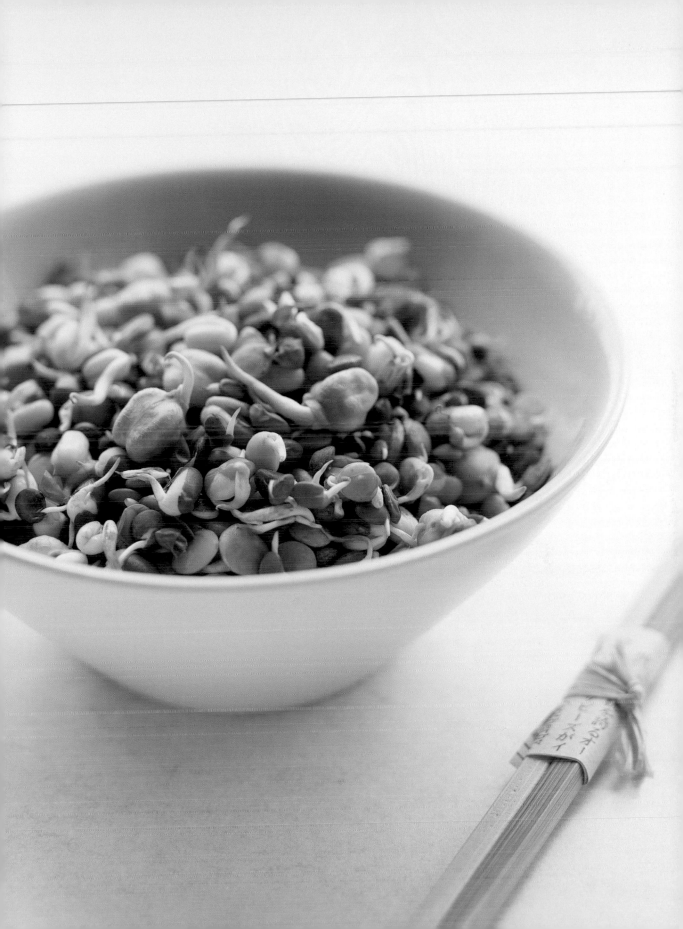

Chickpeas

Chickpeas produce very crisp and sweet sprouts. Harvest after four or five days. Do not allow them to grow too long or they will go woody.

Cress

No soaking required. However, this is a mucilaginous sprout which means that it forms a jelly-like substance while sprouting. Because of this it should not be grown in jars but in earthenware saucers or on blotting paper. Harvest after four or five days.

Fenugreek

Fenugreek seeds produce quite spicy sprouts with a definite flavour. Harvest after three or four days. After this time the flavour tends to diminish.

Flageolet Beans

These produce good crisp and sweet sprouts. Harvest after three to five days.

Haricot Beans

These produce good crisp sprouts. Harvest after three to five days.

Lentils

Use whole lentils and soak them for six to eight hours. They produce distinctive sprouts which are excellent harvested after two or three days. However, they can be left for up to five days.

Millet

This produces a chewy sprout which should be harvested within two or three days.

Mung Beans

These are the most widely sprouted bean. The sprouts remain sweet until they are quite large. Harvest after four to six days.

Mustard

No soaking required. This is a mucilaginous seed which should be grown on earthenware saucers or blotting paper. Produces a spicy sprout which should be harvested after four or five days.

Oats
Use unhulled oats and harvest as soon as the sprout is as long as the seed.

Peas
Use whole dried peas to give a crisp and sweet sprout similar to sprouted chickpeas. Harvest after two or three days or they will become rather tough.

Pumpkin Seeds
These produce very nutty sprouts which should be harvested after three or four days before they start to go bitter. Remove the husks which may be very tough.

Radish Seeds
No soaking required. This is a mucilaginous seed which should be grown in earthenware saucers or on blotting paper. Produces a tangy, spicy sprout which should be harvested after four or five days.

Sesame
Use unhulled seeds and soak for six to eight hours. Produces sprouts with a distinctive flavour. Harvest after three or four days before they begin to go bitter.

Soya Beans
These can be difficult to sprout so try to buy beans which are not too old. Soak for eight hours and keep in a cool place, as they have a tendency to ferment. Rinse the growing sprouts very regularly and harvest after three to six days.

Sunflower Seeds
Hulled sunflower seeds can be used for sprouting. Provides a very attractive nutty sprout which should be harvested after three or four days before the flavour turns bitter.

Wheat
Use wholegrain, not cracked, wheat. Provides a very sweet sprout which should be harvested after two or three days, when the sprout is about the same length as the seed.

pâtés

It's very useful to have a good home-made pâté in the fridge, to serve on oatcakes, crackers or rye or as a quick snack or to offer as a ready-to-serve first course. You can also use it as a topping for canapés and as a sandwich-filler.

quick salmon pâté

Canned salmon works very well in this recipe but if you ever have any freshly poached salmon left over from a meal it makes an even more luxurious pâté.

ingredients

1 x 213g (7½oz) can red salmon, well drained
100g (3½oz) smoked salmon pieces
175g (6oz) low-fat curd or cottage cheese or silken tofu
juice of ½ lemon
plenty of freshly ground black pepper

method

1 Flake the tinned salmon into a blender, removing the skin if you prefer not to have dark flecks in the pâté. Leave the bones to be ground into the mix.

2 Add the smoked salmon, the cheese or tofu, lemon juice and black pepper, and blend until smooth.

3 Spoon into a small container and cover with a lid. Store in the fridge until required.

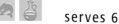 **serves 6**

egg and onion pâté

This pâté does not keep for quite so long in the fridge as some of the others and it cannot be frozen. If you are allergic to eggs you can replace them with mashed goat's cheese. Serve with celery and cucumber sticks.

ingredients
4 free-range eggs
4–6 small spring onions, finely chopped
50g (2oz) watercress, finely chopped
freshly ground black pepper (to taste)
1–1½ tablespoons low-fat natural live yoghurt

method **1** Hard-boil the eggs and leave to cool. Shell them and mash with a fork. Stir in all the remaining ingredients, adding sufficient yoghurt to give a good consistency. Chill before using.

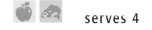 serves 4

raw mushroom pâté

I sometimes make this well-flavoured pâté with Feta cheese and sometimes with tofu. The taste is much sharper and saltier if you use Feta. Serve it with rye bread.

ingredients
100g (3½oz) shiitake mushrooms, washed and trimmed
100g (3½oz) Feta cheese or ordinary tofu
5–6 small spring onions, trimmed and chopped
2 tablespoons freshly chopped parsley
freshly ground black pepper (to taste)
a pinch of salt (if using tofu)

method **1** Place all the ingredients in a blender and process until very smooth.

2 Spoon the pâté into a small container. Cover and keep it in the fridge until required.

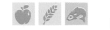 serves 2

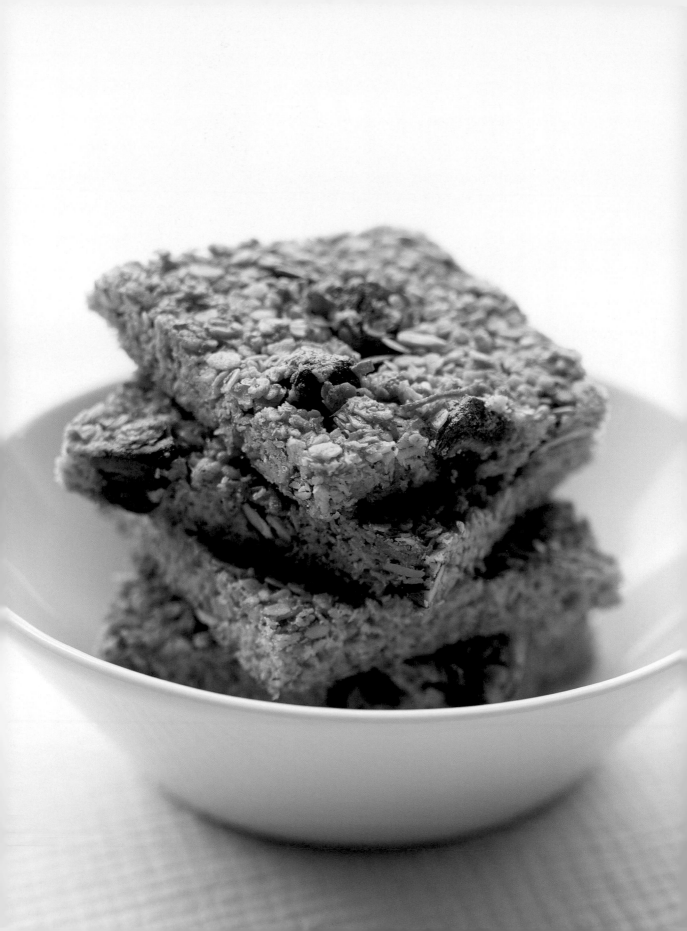

biscuits and cakes

seed and coconut flapjack

If you cannot find brown rice syrup you can use any other syrup or even a mixture of syrup and honey.

ingredients

150g (5½oz) porridge oats
2 tablespoons desiccated coconut
1 tablespoon sunflower seeds
1 tablespoon pumpkin seeds, roughly chopped
1 tablespoon linseeds
25g (1oz) chopped dates (optional)
3 tablespoons brown rice syrup
5 tablespoons cold-pressed walnut oil

method

1 Set the oven to 180°C/350°F/Gas 4.

2 Mix all the dry ingredients together. Add the syrup and oil and mix very well to ensure an even distribution.

3 Press into a lightly greased 14 x 14cm (5½ x 5½in) tin and bake for about 25–30 minutes. Cut into fingers and leave to cool in the tin.

2 slices =   **makes about 8 slices**

lexia raisin flapjack

This is quite a soft flapjack and it makes a great addition to lunchboxes for adults and kids alike. However, if you want a crunchier flapjack, try Seed and Coconut Flapjack (see page 93).

ingredients

300g (10½oz) lexia raisins, washed and dried

75ml (3fl oz) extra-virgin olive oil

250g (9oz) rolled oats

50g (2oz) desiccated coconut

1 tablespoon malt extract (optional)

method

1 Set the oven to 180°C/350°F/Gas 4.

2 Place the raisins in a pan with 150ml (5fl oz) water and heat gently for about 10 minutes to soften them. Cool slightly.

3 Place the contents of the pan in a food processor and process briefly. Stir in the olive oil, oats, coconut and malt, if using, and mix well together.

4 Press this mixture into a 27 × 18cm (7 × 11in) Swiss roll tin and smooth over the top. Place in the oven and bake for 20–25 minutes until lightly browned on top. Cool in the tin.

2 slices = **makes 12–14 slices**

sesame biscuits

If you have a problem with gluten simply substitute half-and-half soya flour and brown rice flour for the wholemeal flour.

ingredients

50g (2oz) unsalted butter

100g (3½oz) wholemeal flour

25g (1oz) fine oatmeal

25g (1oz) sesame seeds

25g (1oz) sunflower seeds

2–3 tablespoons soya or rice milk

method   **1** Set the oven to 190°C/375°F/Gas 5 and line a baking tray with baking parchment.

2 Rub the butter into the flour and oatmeal and stir in the seeds. Then use the milk to bind the mixture. Use 2 tablespoons to start with, adding more milk as necessary until the mixture forms a moist ball.

3 Place on a floured board and roll out to about 0.3cm (1/8 in) thick. (If you roll the mixture too thinly it will be impossible to cut into shapes.)

4 Use a fluted cutter to make 5–6cm (2–2¼ in) rounds and place on the prepared tray. Place in the oven and bake for 15 minutes. Cool on a wire rack.

2 biscuits = **makes 10–12 biscuits**

sesame pitta sticks

These crisp pitta sticks are excellent made with extra-virgin olive oil or with butter. Serve on their own or with dips and pâtés.

ingredients
    2 wholemeal pitta breads
    2 tablespoons extra-virgin olive oil or melted butter
    3 tablespoons sesame seeds

method   **1** Set the oven to 230°C/450°F/Gas 8.

2 Brush the pitta breads on both sides with olive oil or melted butter. Place on a baking tray and sprinkle thickly with the sesame seeds.

3 Cut into long thin strips and bake for about 4–5 minutes until crisp and golden, taking care not to let them burn.

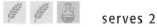 **serves 2**

sunflower seed and carrot muffins

The sunflower seeds give these special occasion muffins quite a crunchy texture. If you like a smoother texture, roughly chop the seeds before you add them.

ingredients

150g (5½oz) brown rice flour
75g (3oz) fine oatmeal
1 level tablespoon baking powder
½ teaspoon ground cinnamon
¼ teaspoon salt
2 large eggs
175ml (6fl oz) milk
2 tablespoons cold-pressed mixed seed oil
100g (3½oz) carrots, coarsely grated
75g (3oz) raisins
50g (2oz) sunflower seeds

method

1 Set the oven to 190°C/375°F/Gas 5 and grease a bun or muffin tray.

2 Mix the flour and oatmeal with the baking powder, cinnamon and salt. Beat the eggs with the milk and oil. Stir the carrots, raisins and sunflower seeds into the dry ingredients and add the egg mixture. Fold the mixture well and spoon into the prepared bun or muffin tray.

3 Bake the muffins for 25 minutes, then turn out onto a wire rack to cool.

2 muffins =   **makes 10–12**

soups

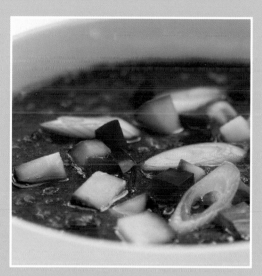

stock

A good stock is essential for a good soup and today you can buy excellent preservative- and additive-free stocks, bouillon cubes or pastes made from chicken, fish or vegetables. Some of them are also made from organic ingredients.

However, ready-made stocks are quite expensive and it is easy to make your own at home. Just gather the ingredients together and boil them up in quantity at the same time as you are cooking a meal. When the stock is made, store it in the fridge or in the freezer in boxes of various sizes. You should also freeze some in ice cube trays so that you will have small quantities available for braising or making sauces.

Make an effort, too, to keep any liquor that remains after steaming or boiling vegetables. This can be used as it is, or boiled up with more vegetable peelings, discarded lettuce leaves or watercress stalks to make a simple stock. Yeast extracts can also help to pep up vegetable stocks, but take care not to use too much, as most of them have very specific flavours which might take over in a recipe.

If you roast a whole chicken or any other bird, you should always boil up the left-over carcass afterwards to make a good poultry stock. Some butchers will sell you raw chicken carcasses from chickens which have been cut up for breast fillets and these give an even more flavoursome result.

If you are buying fish, ask the fishmonger to give you the head and the bones to boil up for fish stock. Avoid the skin, as this can give a rather gelatinous texture.

The following recipes make about 1 litre (1¾ pints) of three basic stocks. If you need a stronger stock for a particular recipe, simply boil up the basic stock to reduce the quantity and intensify the flavour.

vegetable stock

You can, of course, add any bits and pieces of old vegetables which you happen to have to hand but it's best to avoid broccoli, cabbage, sprouts, parsnips and celeriac. These have a very specific flavour which you may not want in a stock for general use.

ingredients

1 large onion, trimmed but not peeled
1 leek, trimmed
2 carrots, washed but not peeled
2 sticks celery
1 bay leaf
a few sprigs of fresh parsley

1 Chop all the vegetables up into fairly small pieces to extract the most flavour, and then place them in a large saucepan with 1.4 litres (2¹/₂ pints) water and the herbs.

2 Cover with a lid and bring to the boil. Simmer for about 40–45 minutes, stirring from time to time. The liquor should reduce to about 1 litre (1³/₄ pints). Strain well and store.

fish stock

Choose white fish heads and bones from cod, haddock, whiting, brill, mullet and sea bass (rather than oily fish such as herring or mackerel which will give too strong a flavour).

ingredients
2 fish heads and plenty of bones
2 carrots, peeled and chopped
1 onion, peeled and chopped
1 bay leaf
a few sprigs of parsley

method **1** Place all the ingredients in a large saucepan with 1.2 litres (2 pints) water and bring to the boil. Cover with a lid and simmer for half an hour.

2 Strain through muslin and store.

chicken stock

ingredients
2 raw chicken carcasses or 1 small chicken leg joint
1 large onion, trimmed but not peeled
1 carrot, peeled
1 stick celery
1 bay leaf

method **1** Place the chicken carcasses or leg joint in a large casserole and cover with 1.4 litres (2¹/₂ pints) water. Add all the remaining ingredients and bring to the boil. Cover and simmer for one hour, breaking up the carcass or joint with a wooden spoon after about half an hour.

2 Strain well and store.

gazpacho

Choose the ripest and most flavoursome tomatoes you can find for this famous Andalucian soup. If you are not sure of the quality of your tomatoes, add some good tomato purée.

ingredients

225g (8oz) ripe tomatoes, roughly chopped
1 large clove of garlic, peeled and chopped
4–5 spring onions, trimmed and chopped
½ red pepper, seeded and chopped
5cm (2in) length cucumber, roughly chopped
225ml (8fl oz) passata
juice of 1 lemon
1½ tablespoons extra-virgin olive oil
salt and freshly ground black pepper (to taste)

GARNISH
2.5cm (1in) cucumber, diced
¼ red or green pepper, seeded and diced
1 tablespoon freshly chopped spring onions

method

1 Place the tomatoes in a blender with the garlic and process for a minute. Add the rest of the vegetables and process again. Take care not to over-process – the soup should have quite a rough texture.

2 Transfer to a bowl and stir in the rest of the soup ingredients. Leave to stand in the fridge for 15–20 minutes. Prepare the cucumber, pepper and spring onion for the Garnish and serve sprinkled over the soup.

serves 2

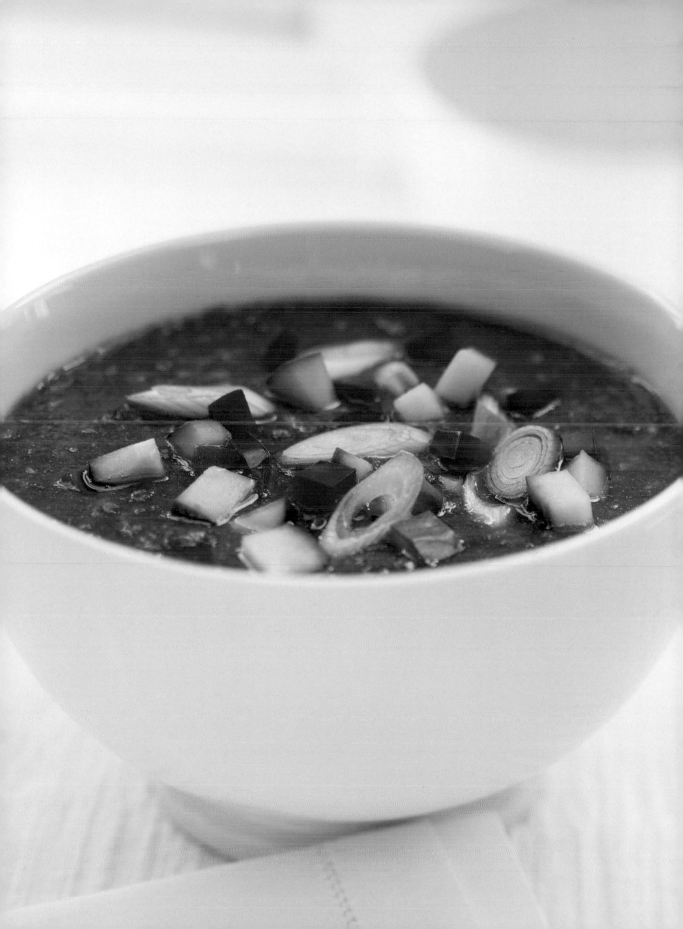

energy soup

This thick, raw-style soup offers instant high energy coupled with plenty of vitamins and minerals. You can give it a subtle change of flavour by adding chopped fresh herbs such as parsley, chervil, mint, coriander or basil. Serve with oatcakes or rice cakes.

ingredients

225g (8oz) carrots, peeled and roughly chopped
3–4 broccoli florets
½ bunch watercress
100g (3½oz) firm tofu
3 teaspoons stock concentrate
1 teaspoon tomato purée
75–100ml (3–3½fl oz) soya milk

method

1 Place all the ingredients in a blender and process well. Add soya milk until you get the consistency you prefer.

2 Serve cold or gently heat, without letting the soup boil.

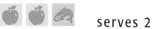 serves 2

green root soup

Joanna Kjaer, author of Beat Candida Through Diet, *has created this deliciously velvety, green soup to suit everyone. It is gluten-free, dairy-free, yeast-free and egg-free. She suggests that you use organic vegetables and grate the skins with the flesh.*

ingredients

3 tablespoons cold-pressed organic sunflower oil
75g (3oz) potatoes, scrubbed and grated
50g (2oz) Jerusalem artichokes, scrubbed and grated
50g (2oz) leeks, finely sliced
40g (1½oz) watercress
15g (½oz) parsley
sea salt and black pepper (to taste)

method   **1** Heat the oil in a large saucepan and add the grated potatoes and artichokes. Cook over a moderate heat for a few minutes and then add half the leeks, watercress and parsley. Continue to cook gently until the greens wilt.

2 Add 300ml (10fl oz) water to the pan and bring to the boil. Reduce the heat and simmer for another 5 minutes or so until the potatoes and artichokes are cooked through.

3 Transfer to a blender and process until thick and creamy.

4 Return to the pan, heat through and season to taste. Pour into bowls and top with the rest of the leeks, watercress and parsley, finely chopped.

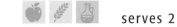 **serves 2**

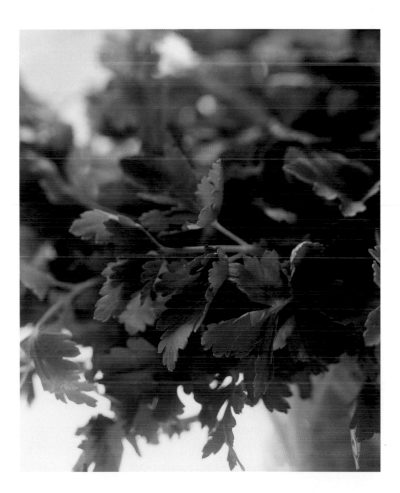

celery and apple soup with ginger

This is another raw-style hot soup which can also be served chilled on hot summer days. Add a dollop of Greek yoghurt to the chilled version and serve with Sesame Pitta Sticks (see page 95).

In the winter you can use a small leek in place of the spring onions.

ingredients

150g (5½oz) eating apples, cored and chopped

150g (5½oz) celery, thinly sliced

3–5 spring onions, trimmed and chopped

1cm (½in) slice of fresh root ginger, peeled and grated

225ml (8fl oz) vegetable stock

method

1 Place all the ingredients in a food professor and blend to a purée.

2 Transfer to a small saucepan, warm gently over a low heat and serve.

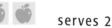

serves 2

avocado and green bean broth

You'll love the contrasting textures of the velvety avocado and the slightly crunchy green beans in this unusual soup from California. If the weather is hot you can have it chilled, adding the avocado and lemon juice just before serving.

ingredients

500ml (16fl oz) good vegetable or chicken stock

100g (3½oz) green beans, trimmed and cut in half

2 spring onions, coarsely chopped

½ ripe avocado, pitted, peeled and sliced

juice of ½ lemon

3–4 drops Tabasco sauce (optional)

method **1** Place the stock in a pan with the green beans and bring to the boil. Cook for 5–6 minutes until the beans are slightly softened but still firm to the bite.

2 Add all the remaining ingredients and serve at once.

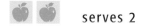 **serves 2**

carrot soup in the raw

Ever had a raw, hot soup? This soup is blended cold and then heated gently, keeping all the vitamin and mineral content intact. It's also full of fibre. Don't overheat it or you will defeat the object.

ingredients

225g (8oz) carrots, peeled and roughly chopped
1 spring onion, trimmed and chopped
40g (1½oz) ground almonds
175ml (6fl oz) soya or skimmed milk
1 tablespoon freshly chopped mixed herbs or ½ teaspoon dried mixed herbs

method **1** Place the carrots in a food processor with the spring onion and blend to a purée. Add all the other ingredients and process until well mixed.

2 Transfer to a small saucepan, warm gently over a low heat and serve.

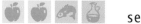 **serves 2**

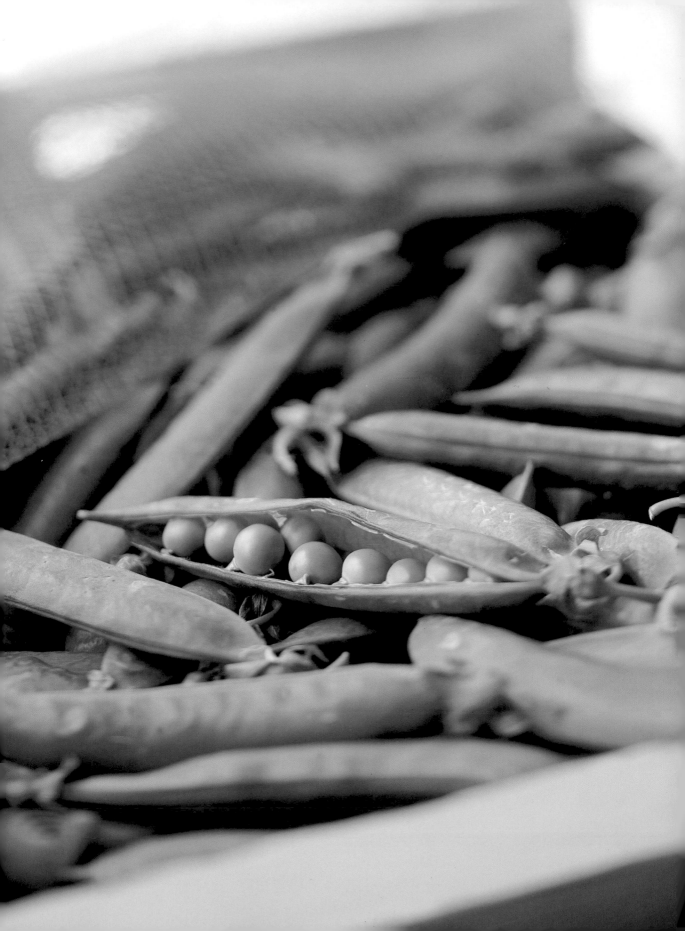

chilled cucumber soup with fresh mint and peas

Always use fresh rather than dried mint. The latter has a very bitter flavour which is not true to the fresh herb. Frozen chopped mint is quite good if the fresh herb is not available.

ingredients

2 small cucumbers, grated
150g (5½oz) low-fat natural live yoghurt
2–3 tablespoons freshly chopped mint
50g (2oz) very small fresh peas or cooked frozen peas
100ml (4fl oz) good vegetable stock
freshly ground black pepper (to taste)
a little paprika pepper
a few sprigs of fresh mint

method

1 Mix the grated cucumber with the yoghurt, mint and peas in a large bowl and stir in the stock. Season with black pepper.

2 Chill in the fridge for as long as you can before serving.

3 Serve garnished with a little paprika pepper sprinkled over the top and some sprigs of fresh mint.

serves 2

broccoli and sprouted sunflower seed soup

If you like a chunky, crunchy soup, simply add the sunflower seed sprouts as soon as the broccoli has softened and serve at once. Alternatively, purée the soup in a blender and then add the beansprouts or purée the whole lot! The choice is yours.

ingredients

½ onion, peeled and chopped
1 small carrot, peeled and chopped
250g (9oz) head of broccoli, broken into florets
freshly ground black pepper (to taste)
100g (3½oz) sprouted sunflower seeds

method

1 Place the onion, carrot and broccoli in a large pan and add 700ml (23fl oz) water and black pepper. Bring to the boil and reduce the heat. Simmer for 15–20 minutes, or less if you have cut the vegetables into small pieces.

2 Add the sprouted sunflower seeds and serve the soup either as it is or puréed.

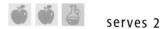

serves 2

miso soup with tofu

The best miso soup is made with a good miso paste but if you do not do very much Japanese cooking it can be difficult to use up the paste before it goes off. One answer is to use a packet of instant miso soup. This gives you a chance to try out a new flavour without learning a lot of new techniques.

ingredients

2 teaspoons cold-pressed mixed seed oil
1 onion, peeled and thinly sliced
1 teaspoon freshly grated root ginger
100g (3½oz) mangetout or small courgettes, sliced
100g (3½oz) deep-fried tofu, cut in half
2 single-serving packets of instant miso soup
6–8 spring onions, sliced diagonally

method   **1**   Heat the oil in a saucepan and gently sweat the onion and ginger for 3–4 minutes. Do not allow the onion to brown. Add the mangetout or courgettes, tofu and 500ml (16fl oz) boiling water and bring back to the boil. Simmer for a further 2–3 minutes.

  2   Spoon the tofu and vegetables into two soup bowls. Pour the liquor over the instant miso soup mix and stir well. Then pour the soup over the vegetables and garnish with the spring onion. Serve at once.

 **serves 2**

sweet potato and carrot soup

This wonderfully creamy soup couldn't be easier to make. Its bright orange colour reflects the high level of carotenoids in these year-round vegetables. A good alternative to sweet potato is butternut squash.

ingredients   250g (9oz) sweet potatoes, peeled and finely chopped
     250g (9oz) carrots, scrubbed and finely chopped
     100ml (3½fl oz) canned coconut milk
     ½–1 clove garlic (to taste), crushed
     black pepper (to taste)

method   **1**   Boil the sweet potatoes and carrots in 350ml (12fl oz) water for about 15 minutes until soft.

  2   Purée the soup in a blender with the coconut milk, garlic and black pepper, then serve.

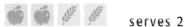 **serves 2**

hot sour prawn soup

Tamarind paste gives this South-East Asian soup a deep lemony flavour. You can buy tamarind in ethnic grocers and some specialist delicatessens. If you cannot find it, try lemon juice.

ingredients

600ml (1 pint) chicken stock
½ teaspoon tamarind paste
1 small fresh green chilli
1 dried red chilli
1 piece lemon grass
2 slices fresh lime
2 small carrots, peeled and sliced diagonally
75g (3oz) broccoli, broken into small florets
50g (2oz) pak choy or Chinese greens, coarsely sliced
4–6 spring onions, sliced diagonally
1 tablespoon soy sauce
4–6 large King prawns, cooked and peeled
plenty of fresh coriander leaves

method

1 Pour the stock into a saucepan and add the tamarind paste, chillies, lemon grass and lime. Bring to the boil and simmer for about 10–15 minutes.

2 Prepare the vegetables, add the carrots and broccoli to the pan and continue to simmer for a further 2–3 minutes.

3 Now add all the remaining ingredients except the coriander. Return to the boil and serve garnished with plenty of fresh coriander leaves.

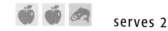 serves 2

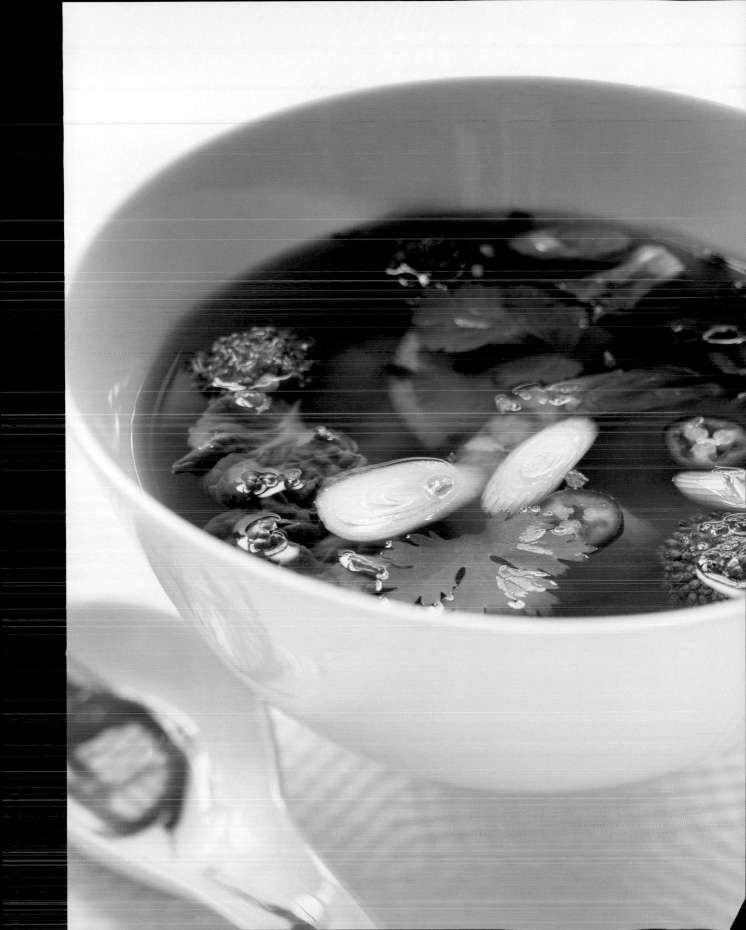

ginger, chicken and beansprout soup

There's no need to add chilli to a dish to make it hot and spicy. Freshly grated ginger and black pepper work just as well, which is good news if you react adversely to chilli peppers.

ingredients

1 medium onion, peeled and roughly chopped

1 large chicken drumstick, skinned

2.5cm (1in) fresh root ginger, peeled and grated

2 cloves of garlic, peeled and roughly chopped

½ medium red pepper, seeded and cut into strips

6 spring onions, trimmed and roughly chopped

2 teaspoons dark soy sauce

75g (3oz) mung beansprouts

freshly ground black pepper (to taste)

juice of ½ lemon

method

1 Place the onion in a saucepan with the chicken drumstick and 800ml (28fl oz) water. Add half the ginger and one clove of garlic. Bring to the boil, reduce the heat and simmer for about 30 minutes, until the chicken is cooked through and the stock has reduced to about 600ml (1 pint).

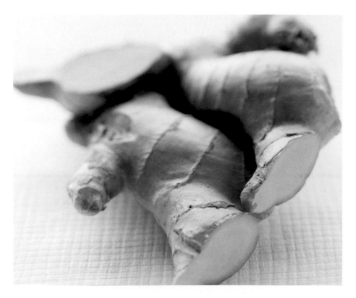

2 Remove the cooked drumstick from the pan and set to one side. Strain the liquid from the pan into another saucepan, discarding the onion. Remove the cooked chicken meat from the bone and add to the pan with the cooking liquor.

3 Return the soup to the boil and add the red pepper, spring onions, remaining ginger and garlic and the soy sauce. Cook for 2–3 minutes, before adding the beansprouts, black pepper and lemon juice. Heat through for a minute or so and serve at once.

serves 2

spicy lentil and watercress soup

By adding the watercress to the soup at the very last minute you will get every bit of benefit from its nutrients. Put it all in — even the long stalks.

ingredients

50g (2oz) red split lentils, picked over and washed
1 small onion, peeled and chopped
1 small carrot, peeled and chopped
600ml (1 pint) vegetable stock or water
1 bay leaf
½ teaspoon mild curry powder
¼ teaspoon dried thyme
¼ teaspoon celery salt
freshly ground black pepper (to taste)
50g (2oz) watercress

method

1 Place all the ingredients except the watercress in a saucepan and bring to the boil. Cover with a lid, reduce the heat and simmer for 30 minutes.

2 Remove the bay leaf and purée in a blender. Add the watercress, whizz quickly and reheat. Serve at once.

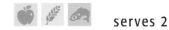 **serves 2**

chunky bean and kale soup

This main course soup is excellent poured over a hunk of day-old bread in the Tuscan manner. Alternatively, you can serve it over toasted polenta squares or with rye bread. Finish off the meal with Hunza Apricots and Cashew Cream (see page 201).

ingredients

1 teaspoon extra-virgin olive oil

1 medium onion, peeled and chopped

2 sticks celery, sliced

1 carrot, peeled and diced

500ml (16fl oz) well-flavoured vegetable stock

150g (5½oz) cooked or canned red kidney beans

150g (5½oz) curly kale, shredded

1 tablespoon tomato purée

½ teaspoon dried oregano

1 clove garlic, peeled and finely chopped

salt and freshly ground black pepper (to taste)

method

1 Heat the oil in a large saucepan and add all the fresh vegetables except the kale. Stir over a very low heat for 2–3 minutes to release all the flavours.

2 Add the stock and bring to the boil. Reduce the heat and cook for 15 minutes.

3 Mash half the kidney beans with a potato masher and add to the soup with the whole beans, the shredded kale, tomato purée, herbs and seasonings and continue cooking for another 10 minutes. Very tough kale may need a little longer to soften.

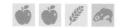 serves 2

starters

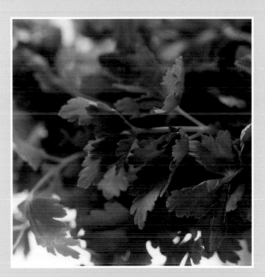

cold starters

rocket salad with chickpeas in tahini dressing

You can use any bitter leaves for this spicy salad. Try it with the cultivated dandelion leaves you can often buy at Greek delis or with watercress or even mustard and cress.

ingredients

a handful of rocket, approximately 25g (1oz)
3–4 large sprigs broadleaf parsley
100g (3½oz) canned chickpeas, drained weight
½ red pepper, seeded and very finely chopped

TAHINI DRESSING
1 heaped teaspoon tahini paste
2 teaspoons cold-pressed mixed seed oil
1 teaspoon lemon juice

method

1 Arrange the rocket and parsley on two small plates or shallow entrée dishes and sprinkle with the chickpeas and chopped red pepper.

2 Mix all the Tahini Dressing ingredients together in a cup with 2 teaspoons water and spoon a little over each salad. Serve at once.

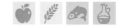

serves 2

grilled pepper ramekins with guacamole

You can really cheat with this recipe by buying ready-prepared guacamole, but we think home-made is best!

ingredients

2 large red peppers
a few rocket leaves (to garnish)

GUACAMOLE
1 small avocado
juice of 1 lemon
2 tablespoons freshly chopped coriander
1 clove garlic, crushed

method

1 Cut the peppers into large pieces and remove the seeds. Place under a hot grill until well seared. Leave to cool and then remove the skins.

2 Place all the Guacamole ingredients in a blender and process until smooth. If you like a chunkier texture, mash the avocado with a fork and stir in the remaining ingredients.

3 Line two ramekin dishes with the grilled peppers, retaining some for the top. Spoon the avocado mixture into the centre and top with the remaining peppers.

4 Place in the fridge to chill before turning out to serve. Garnish with rocket.

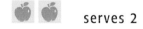 **serves 2**

grilled aubergines with fresh mint

This is such a simple dish but the flavours are stunning. Serve with some good bread to soak up the juices.

ingredients

1 aubergine, cut into about 12 slices

3 tablespoons extra-virgin olive oil

4–6 sprigs of fresh mint

1 teaspoon dried oregano

a little salt and freshly ground black pepper (to taste)

method

1 Brush the slices of aubergine very lightly with olive oil and place under a hot grill. Cook for 2–3 minutes on each side until lightly browned and cooked through.

2 Place four slices of aubergine on a shallow platter and top each one with some mint leaves, oregano and seasoning. Cover with another slice of aubergine and repeat the process, finishing with the final layer of aubergine.

3 Drizzle the remaining olive oil over each mound and leave on one side to cool, turning the mounds over from time to time.

serves 2

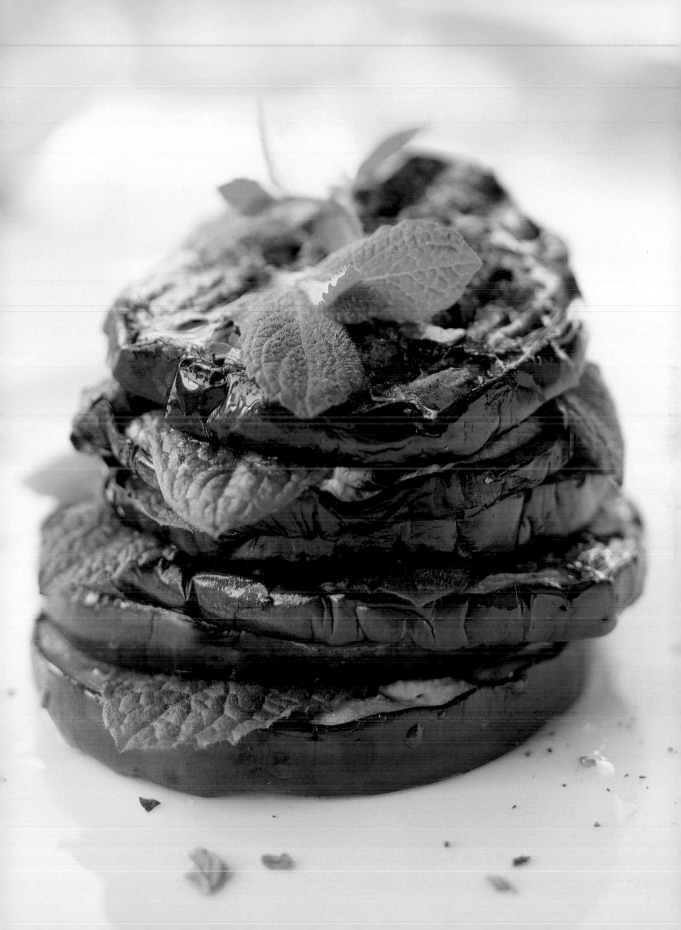

aubergine and grilled pepper terrine

This wonderful vegetable terrine from Italy uses quite a lot of olive oil but it is a special occasion dish which serves four people. Vegetarians can substitute fresh herbs such as tarragon or basil for the anchovies.

ingredients

2 large aubergines, sliced lengthways
75ml (3fl oz) olive oil, plus extra for brushing
4 red peppers, seeded and cut into large pieces
3–4 anchovies, crushed
3 cloves garlic, peeled and crushed
salt and freshly ground black pepper (to taste)

method

1 Brush the aubergine slices with a little olive oil and grill on both sides until lightly golden. Keep on one side.

2 Grill the peppers until the skin darkens. Leave to cool and remove the charred skin.

3 Place the rest of the olive oil in a small saucepan with the rest of the ingredients. Heat gently and then let it sizzle for 2–3 minutes. Take care not to let it burn.

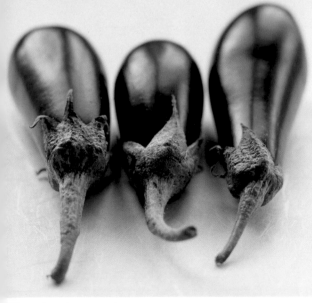

4 Preheat the oven to 180°C/350°F/Gas 4, and brush a 450g (1lb) ovenproof pyrex loaf tin with oil. Line the base and sides with some of the aubergine slices, retaining some for the top. Add half the peppers.

5 Beat the warm oil and anchovy mixture with a fork and pour half of it over the peppers. Repeat with the rest of the peppers and the oil mixture and cover with the retained aubergine slices.

6 Cover with foil and bake for 30 minutes. Remove from the oven and place weights on top of the terrine. Leave to cool and then place in the fridge until required. Turn out to serve and cut into slices.

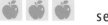

serves 4

bulgarian salad with feta cheese

This simple but very effective starter appears on the menu at almost every Bulgarian restaurant, hence the title.

ingredients

2 tomatoes
1 small cucumber
1 red or green pepper
4 spring onions, chopped
3 tablespoons freshly chopped mint
freshly ground black pepper (to taste)
juice of 1 lemon
75g (3oz) Feta cheese, crumbled

method

1 Cut the tomatoes, cucumber and pepper into very small dice and mix with the chopped spring onions and mint, retaining a few sprigs for decoration. Spoon the mixture into two bowls.

2 Sprinkle with black pepper and lemon juice. Top with the Feta cheese and serve decorated with the retained sprigs of mint.

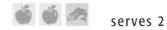 serves 2

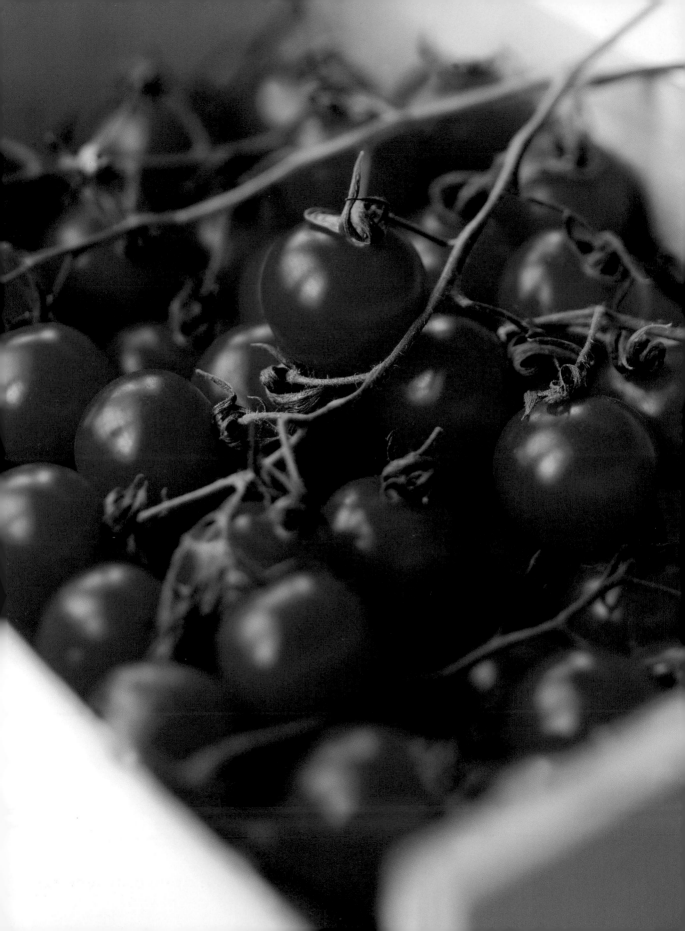

tomato salad with green lentils and sesame tofu dressing

The best green lentils come either from Puy in the Auvergne or from Castelluccio di Norcia in Umbria. Both these products have DOP (or denomination of origin status), which means that the lentils must come from the designated areas, and both varieties are very small and sweet.

ingredients

35g (1¼oz) whole green lentils
2 large Continental tomatoes, sliced

SESAME TOFU DRESSING
100g (3½oz) tofu
50ml (2fl oz) soya milk
1 clove garlic, crushed
1 tablespoon tahini
juice of ½ small lemon
½–1 teaspoon soy sauce (to taste)

method

1 Place the lentils in a saucepan and cover with 100ml (3½fl oz) water. Bring to the boil, cover and simmer over a low heat for 20–25 minutes until the lentils are almost cooked, but still *al dente*. Drain and leave to cool.

2 Place all the dressing ingredients in a blender and process quickly until the consistency is smooth and fairly runny.

3 Arrange the sliced tomatoes on individual plates and scatter the cooked lentils over the top. Spoon on the Sesame Tofu Dressing and serve.

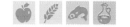

serves 2

tuna and tapenade stuffed tomatoes

This is a really quick and easy starter which comes straight from a well-stocked store cupboard. You can use green or black olive tapenade (available at many supermarkets) but do choose one with plenty of garlic in it.

ingredients

1 x 100g (3½oz) can tuna in oil, drained
2 spring onions, trimmed and finely chopped
75g (3oz) olive tapenade
2 large Continental tomatoes
a few sprigs of fresh parsley

method

1 Mix the tuna with the spring onions and tapenade.

2 Cut the tops off the tomatoes and scoop out the centres and seeds. Chop up the lids and the bits from the centre and add to the tuna mix.

3 Pile the mixture back into the hollowed-out tomatoes garnish with plenty of parsley and serve.

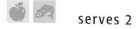 **serves 2**

piquant broccoli salad

Here's an excellent way of eating more of that wonderfully healthy vegetable – broccoli. If you want to maximise the vitamin content, cut out the blanching process. However, the broccoli will be quite hard and you will need to chop it finely before adding the dressing.

ingredients

1 small head broccoli, approximately 200g (7oz)

DRESSING

3–4 cocktail gherkins or 1 small pickled gherkin, finely chopped

6 spring onions, trimmed and chopped

6 radishes, trimmed and chopped

2 tablespoons cold-pressed mixed seed oil

2 teaspoons cider vinegar

¼ **teaspoon made mustard**

freshly ground black pepper (to taste)

method

1 Plunge the broccoli into boiling water and leave for about a minute. Now plunge into cold water. Drain and leave to cool. Cut into bite-sized pieces and arrange in two salad bowls.

2 Place all the Dressing ingredients in a bowl and mix well with the vegetables, it should be a thick consistency. Spoon over the broccoli and leave to stand until cool before serving.

serves 2

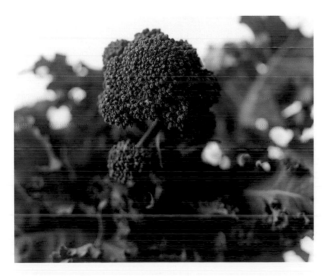

grapefruit and sprouted seed cocktail

This starter has a really fresh and crunchy texture. Add some peeled prawns for special occasions.

ingredients

1 large grapefruit, cut in half
50g (2oz) mung bean sprouts
25g (1oz) sprouted sunflower seeds
¼ red pepper, seeded and finely diced
2 tablespoons freshly chopped parsley
3 tablespoons Greek yoghurt
sprouted alfalfa seeds (to garnish)

method

1 Scoop the flesh out of the grapefruit halves, retaining the skins. Chop the flesh and mix with all the other ingredients, except the alfalfa seeds. Toss well together and spoon the mixture back into the grapefruit skins.

2 Garnish with the alfalfa seeds and serve.

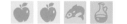 serves 2

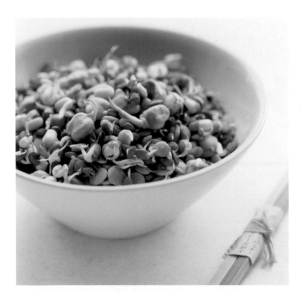

rainbow vegetables with avocado dressing

This is a wonderfully colourful starter with a really fresh taste. It is also very versatile. If you want, you can substitute green, red or yellow peppers, broccoli or cauliflower florets or beansprouts for any of the ingredients specified.

Serve with rye bread or wholemeal rolls.

ingredients

6–8 cherry tomatoes, cut in half
2 sticks celery, cut into diagonal lengths
5cm (2in) length cucumber, cut into thick rounds
6–8 baby carrots, trimmed
a few sprigs of broadleaf parsley

AVOCADO DRESSING
1 small or ½ large avocado, peeled and pitted
½ small clove garlic, crushed
juice of ½ lemon
2 tablespoons low-fat natural live yoghurt
Solo salt and freshly ground black pepper (to taste)

method

1 Start by making the Avocado Dressing. Place all the ingredients in a blender with 2 tablespoons water and process until smooth. Add a little more water if the mixture is too thick.

2 Arrange the vegetables in a colourful pattern on two serving plates. Spoon on the Avocado Dressing and decorate with the sprigs of parsley. Serve at once.

serves 2

hot starters

vegetable samosas with spicy tomato dip

Genuine samosa pastry is difficult to make at home but you can cheat by using filo pastry. The result is deliciously crisp and flaky. Serve single samosas as a first course or two or three as a main course with salad.

ingredients

VEGETABLE SAMOSAS
2 large potatoes, approximately 300g (10oz)
1 tablespoon extra-virgin olive oil, plus extra for brushing
1 teaspoon coriander seeds
½ onion, peeled and chopped
1 teaspoon freshly grated root ginger
50g (2oz) cooked peas
1 green chilli, seeded and chopped
1 teaspoon ground turmeric
½ teaspoon medium curry powder
1 teaspoon lemon juice

12 sheets filo pastry, 30 x 18cm (12 x 7in)

SPICY TOMATO DIP
¼ teaspoon paprika pepper
¼ teaspoon ground cumin
¼ teaspoon ground coriander
2 tablespoons tomato purée
2 teaspoons tomato ketchup
juice of ½ lemon
a little cider vinegar
a little Worcester sauce (optional)

method

1 Preheat the oven to 200°C/400°F/Gas 6. Steam the whole potatoes in their skins – when they are tender, peel and dice.

2 Heat the olive oil in a pan and fry the coriander seeds until they darken. Add the onion and ginger and continue frying until the onion starts to brown and the mixture dries. This will take about 5–6 minutes. Add the potatoes, peas, green chilli, turmeric, curry powder and lemon juice, and mix well together.

3 Brush the filo pastry sheets with olive oil and place two sheets on top of each other. Fold over to form a square. Fill with the potato mixture, folding the pastry into a triangular shape. Seal the edges with a little more oil and place on a baking tray.

4 Repeat until all the pieces of filo have been used up. Bake for 20–25 minutes, turning once or twice until the Samosas are well browned and crisp.

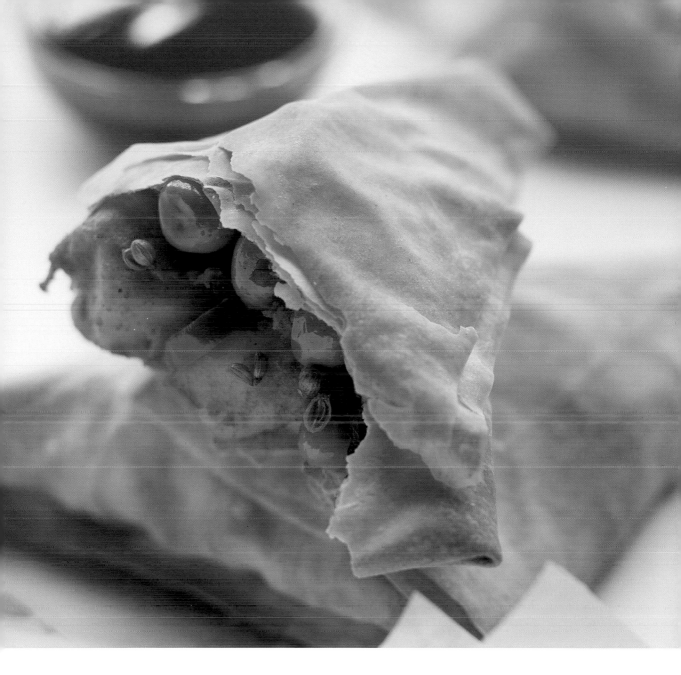

5 Meanwhile to make the Spicy Tomato Dip, mix the spices and toast under the grill on a small piece of foil. Turn frequently to stop them burning.

6 Mix the tomato purée, tomato ketchup and lemon juice together and stir in the toasted spices. Add a little cider vinegar and, if you wish, Worcester sauce to taste. Serve with the Vegetable Samosas.

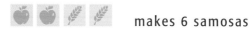 **makes 6 samosas**

smoked tofu on oriental glass noodles with shredded vegetables

This recipe makes an excellent starter, especially for a Thai meal.
Shred the celeriac and carrot by cutting them first into thin slices, then into sticks.

ingredients

600ml (1 pint) good vegetable stock
1 stick lemon grass, cut lengthways down the centre
1 clove of garlic, peeled and sliced
4 thin slices fresh root ginger, peeled
50g (2oz) carrots, peeled
50g (2oz) celeriac, peeled
50g (2oz) Chinese glass noodles or transparent vermicelli
50g (2oz) mangetout
4 spring onions, trimmed and sliced diagonally
3 teaspoons soy sauce
freshly ground black pepper (to taste)
150g/5oz smoked tofu, cut into strips
a few sprigs of fresh coriander

method

1 Put the stock in a large saucepan and add the lemon grass, garlic and ginger. Bring to the boil and simmer for about 10 minutes.

2 Prepare the carrots and celeriac and add to the pan. Continue to cook, uncovered, over a low to medium heat, for a further 3–4 minutes to soften the vegetables.

3 Place the glass noodles or vermicelli in a bowl and pour boiling water over them. Leave to stand for 3–4 minutes. Drain and add to the saucepan with the stock and vegetables. Add the mangetout, spring onions, soy sauce and seasoning and turn up the heat.

4 Boil for a couple of minutes to reduce the sauce a little and ladle into serving bowls. The mixture should be quite runny. Top with smoked tofu and garnish with a few sprigs of fresh coriander.

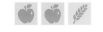

serves 2

stuffed sardines italian-style

Sardines are often over-looked but they, like mackerel and herring, are oily fish with good supplies of Omega 3. This dish from Sicily makes an excellent first course when you are entertaining, and a good lunch too. Ask your fishmonger to split the fish and remove the heads and backbones.

ingredients

6 small or 4 larger sardines, approximately 400g (14oz), gutted

1 slice bread, approximately 40g (1½oz), made into crumbs

40g (1½oz) Parmesan cheese, grated

1 tablespoon freshly chopped parsley

1 teaspoon freshly chopped basil

½ small beaten egg

a knob of butter

2 tablespoons lemon juice

a few sprigs of parsley (to garnish)

lemon wedges (to garnish)

method

1 Wash and prepare the fish if the fishmonger has not done so.

2 Mix the breadcrumbs, Parmesan cheese, parsley and basil with the beaten egg to make a firmish stuffing.

3 Lay the sardines flat, skin side down, and spread with the stuffing. Roll up each fish, starting from the neck end, and fix with half a cocktail stick.

4 Heat the butter in a small shallow pan and arrange the stuffed sardines in the pan. Fry gently for a minute or two, turning once.

5 Then add 4 tablespoons of water and the lemon juice. Cover with a lid and cook for about 10 minutes, turning once again after 5 minutes.

6 Arrange the stuffed sardines on small serving plates and pour on the juices from the pan. Garnish with a few sprigs of parsley and lemon wedges.

 serves 2

twice-baked cheese soufflés
with cucumber and yoghurt sauce

Don't be frightened of making these wonderful little soufflés. They are guaranteed to impress your guests, yet they are really very easy to make.

ingredients
extra-virgin olive oil
plain flour
lightly toasted sesame seeds, ground
25g (1oz) butter
1 level tablespoon plain flour
75ml (3fl oz) milk
75g–100g (3–3½oz) Roquefort or goat's cheese, crumbled or grated
a little nutmeg
salt and pepper (to taste)
3 eggs, separated

CUCUMBER AND YOGHURT SAUCE
6 tablespoons low-fat natural live yoghurt
7cm (3in) length cucumber, diced
salt and pepper (to taste)

method

1 Set the oven to 180°C/350°F/Gas 4.

2 Lightly oil four ramekin dishes and line with a mixture of flour and the sesame seeds.

3 Melt the butter in a saucepan and stir in the flour and milk to make a thick sauce. Cook over a low heat for 2 minutes. Add the cheese, nutmeg and seasonings. Remove from the heat and beat in the egg yolks.

4 Whisk the egg whites until really stiff. Spoon one-third onto the sauce mixture and fold in with a metal spoon. Then fold in the rest of the egg whites.

5 Spoon the mixture into the prepared ramekins, place in a baking tin filled with 2.5cm (1in) boiling water and bake for 20–25 minutes.

6 Remove the ramekins to a wire rack and leave to cool for 10 minutes. Run a spatula round the edges and turn out onto your hand. Place on a greased baking tray.

7 Return the soufflés to the oven for a further 10–15 minutes.

8 Meanwhile, to make the Cucumber and Yoghurt Sauce, mix all the ingredients together in a bowl and serve with the Twice-Baked Cheese Soufflés.

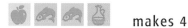

makes 4

grilled scallops on green leaves
with grated celeriac

Buy the freshest scallops you can find and choose spicy rocket or rucola to show off their creamy delicacy. The celeriac adds an extra dimension of creamy aniseed and celery.

ingredients
75g (3oz) rocket or rucola leaves
75g (3oz) peeled celeriac
1 tablespoon lemon juice
2 tablespoons crème fraîche
8 large scallops
a little cold-pressed mixed seed oil
2 lemon wedges

method **1** Arrange the rocket or rucola on two serving plates. Grate the celeriac and mix with the lemon juice and crème fraîche. Place two spoonfuls on each plate.

2 Brush the scallops with a little seed oil and place under a hot grill. Cook for about 2^1/$_2$–3 minutes on each side until they have turned opaque all the way through. Don't overcook.

3 Arrange four scallops on each bed of green leaves, garnish with the lemon wedges and serve at once.

serves 2

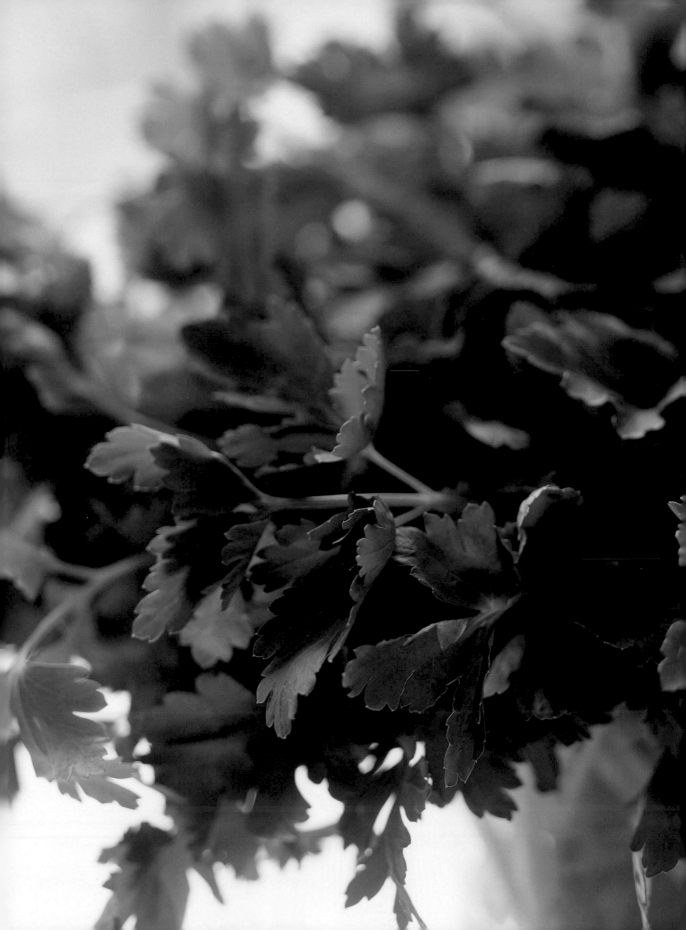

wild mushrooms with kumquats

Unlike oranges, the flesh of kumquats is bitter and the rind is quite sweet. You can, there-fore, just slice and use the whole fruit.

The flavour of these little citrus fruits goes well with most kinds of mushrooms – so you can use whatever you can afford! Here we cheat a little, using dried Italian porcini to give cultivated mushrooms a much more intense flavour.

ingredients

15g (½oz) dried porcini mushrooms

150g (5½oz) mixed cultivated mushrooms, shiitake, brown cap and oyster

2 shallots, peeled and very finely chopped

3–4 kumquats, thinly sliced

a small knob of butter

1 tablespoon extra-virgin olive oil

juice of ½ orange

2 tablespoons freshly chopped parsley

2 large slices rye bread, well toasted

method

1 Pour 4 tablespoons boiling water over the dried porcini and leave to stand for at least half an hour or until required. Remove the mushrooms from the liquor, retaining the latter, and mix with the other mushrooms.

2 Gently sweat the shallots and kumquats in the butter and olive oil for 2–3 minutes to soften a little. Add the mushrooms and toss well.

3 Pour on the liquid from the porcini and the orange juice and bring to the boil. Simmer for 2–3 minutes, adding a little more orange juice or water if required.

4 Add the chopped parsley, spoon the mixture over the toasted rye and serve.

serves 2

spicy tofu satay with peanut sauce and sweetcorn patties

This is another starter for a Thai feast. Make it when you have a little more time. Use the best Thai curry paste you can find, but make your own peanut sauce.

Start by marinating the tofu, then make the sauce and finally the patties. Do not allow the Peanut Sauce to go cold or it may thicken up too much and it can be difficult to thin out again.

ingredients

300g (10oz) deep-fried or firm tofu
2 teaspoons Thai green curry paste
2 tablespoons coconut milk
1 teaspoon Thai fish sauce (optional)

PEANUT SAUCE

1 small onion, very finely chopped
1 clove garlic, peeled and crushed
1 green chilli pepper, seeded and finely chopped
a little very finely chopped lemon grass
1 tablespoon extra-virgin olive oil
75–100ml (3–4fl oz) coconut milk
2 tablespoons wholenut peanut butter

SWEETCORN PATTIES

125g (4½oz) firm tofu
100g (3½oz) sweetcorn
¼ green pepper, seeded and very finely chopped
1 small fresh red chilli pepper, seeded and very finely chopped
½ clove garlic, peeled and crushed
a little freshly grated root ginger
a few drops Thai fish sauce
5–6 tablespoons potato flour
freshly ground black pepper (to taste)
vegetable oil (to fry)

method   **1** Cut the tofu into small cubes and place in a bowl. Mix the remaining ingredients together and spoon over the top of the tofu. Toss well and leave to stand for at least half an hour, turning the tofu in the marinade from time to time.

2 To make the Peanut Sauce, gently sweat the onion, garlic, chilli and lemon grass in the olive oil until well softened. Mash with a potato masher and stir in the coconut milk and peanut butter. Continue stirring over a gentle heat until the sauce is smooth and hot. Add a little more coconut milk if necessary. Keep warm.

3 For the Sweetcorn Patties, mash the tofu with a fork and mix in the sweetcorn with the green pepper, chilli, garlic, ginger and Thai fish sauce. Stir in 3 tablespoons potato flour and some black pepper and mix well. Shape the mixture into eight balls and squeeze them to make the mixture stick together. Carefully flatten each ball and coat on each side in the remaining potato flour. Leave to stand until required.

4 Meanwhile, thread the marinated tofu onto pre-soaked skewers and place under a hot grill for 5–6 minutes, turning from time to time.

5 While the tofu is being grilled, heat about 0.5cm ($^1/_4$ in) vegetable oil in a shallow frying pan and fry the patties on each side until crisp and golden. This will take about 3–4 minutes.

6 Drain the Sweetcorn Patties on kitchen paper and serve immediately with the spicy Tofu Satay and the Peanut Sauce.

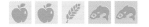

serves 4

warm mushroom and endive salad

These well-flavoured baked mushrooms are served on a bed of curly endive or crinkly frisée. Vegetarians should omit the Worcester sauce and use soy or tamari sauce to pep up the flavour.

ingredients

6 medium or 4 large flat or field mushrooms, approximately 250g (9oz)
2 large cloves garlic, peeled and crushed
1–1½ tablespoons cold-pressed mixed seed oil
1–2 teaspoons Worcester, soy or tamari sauce
freshly ground black pepper (to taste)
3 tablespoons vegetable stock
curly endive or frisée (to serve)
2–3 tablespoons lightly toasted sunflower seeds

method

1 Preheat the oven to 200°C/400°F/Gas 6.

2 Place the mushrooms in an ovenproof dish, gills upward, and spread the crushed garlic over them. Spoon the seed oil and sauce over the mushroom gills and sprinkle with pepper. Spoon the stock into the base of the dish and cover with foil. Bake for about 15–20 minutes until the mushrooms are tender.

3 Arrange the endive or frisée on two serving plates and place the mushrooms on top. Spoon the pan juices over the mushrooms, sprinkle on the lightly toasted sunflower seeds and serve.

 serves 2

main courses

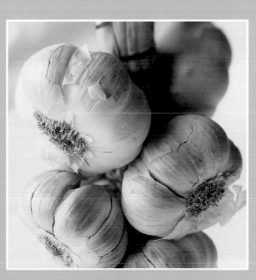

grills

salmon and monkfish kebabs
with coriander and sunflower seed pesto

Here, the Pesto is more of a relish than a sauce. It is quite strong and it lifts this simple rice and fish dish into another dimension.

ingredients

250g (9oz) piece monkfish
250g (9oz) salmon steak
juice of ½ lime
1 teaspoon extra-virgin olive oil
freshly ground black pepper (to taste)
100g (3½oz) rice or quinoa

CORIANDER AND SUNFLOWER SEED PESTO
a bunch of fresh coriander, approximately 25g (1oz)
25g (1oz) sunflower seeds
1 clove garlic, peeled
1 tablespoon cold-pressed mixed seed oil

method

1 Remove the skin and bones from the two fish and cut each one into six large chunks. Thread onto skewers. Mix the lime juice, oil and black pepper and pour evenly over the kebabs. Leave to stand until required for cooking.

2 Cook the rice or quinoa as suggested on page 37.

3 To make the Pesto, place the coriander, sunflower seeds and garlic in a food processor and process quickly. Do not allow the mixture to get too fine. Moisten with the cold-pressed seed oil and keep to one side.

4 Place the kebabs under a hot grill for 2½–3 minutes on each side until just cooked through. Do not allow the fish to overcook or it will be hard and unpleasant. Serve with the rice or quinoa and the Pesto.

serves 2

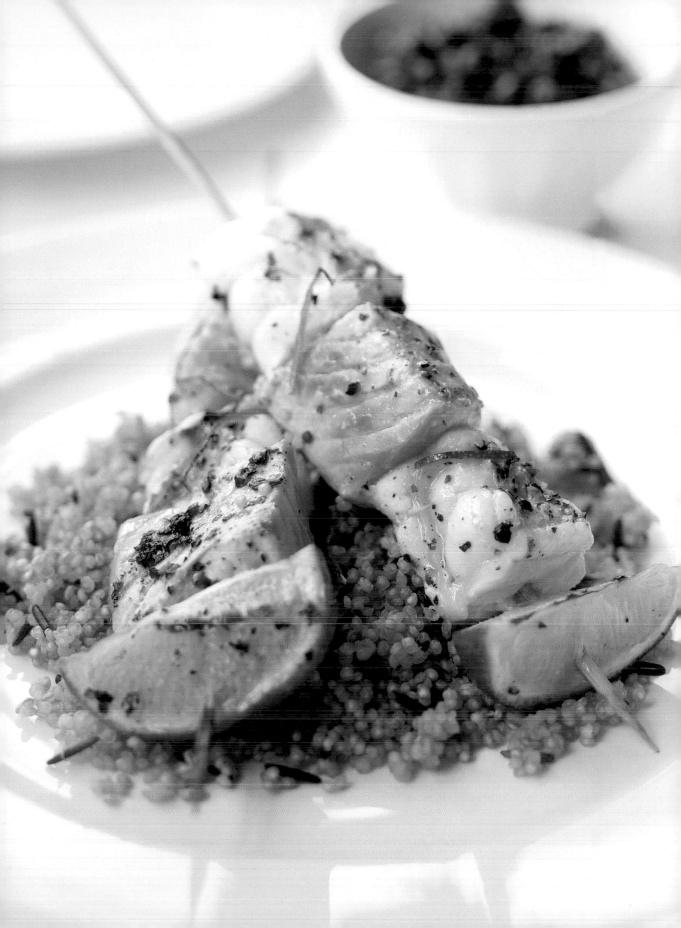

roasted chicory and courgettes with salsa picante and bulgar

If you can find it, you can use Italian red radicchio in place of one of the heads of chicory to give more colour to this delicious roasted vegetable dish.

ingredients

3 large heads of chicory
3 large or 5–6 small courgettes
a little extra-virgin olive oil
cooked bulgar

SALSA PICANTE
1 hard-boiled egg, finely chopped
2 tablespoons freshly chopped parsley
2 tablespoons freshly chopped chives
2 tablespoons capers, finely chopped
2 small green chillies, seeded and finely chopped
juice of ½ small lemon
2–3 tablespoons cold-pressed mixed seed oil

method

1 Cut each head of chicory into three pieces lengthways. Trim and slice the courgettes lengthways. Brush the vegetables with a little olive oil and place the chicory under a hot grill.

2 After 5 minutes, cover the tips of the chicory with a strip of foil to stop the leaves burning and add the courgette slices. Cook for another 8–10 minutes, turning the vegetables from time to time until lightly browned.

3 In the meantime, place all the Salsa ingredients in a bowl and mix well. When the vegetables are cooked, transfer to serving plates with the cooked bulgar. Spoon the Salsa over the top.

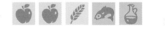

serves 2

vegetarian kebabs with barbecue sauce and brown rice

These vegetable kebabs cook just as well on the barbecue as under the grill.

ingredients

200g (7oz) deep-fried or marinated tofu
1 red pepper, seeded and cut into eight pieces
2 courgettes, thickly sliced
2 small heads fennel, cut into quarters
12 mushrooms
a little extra-virgin olive oil
cooked brown rice (to serve 2)

BARBECUE SAUCE
1 x 200g (7oz) can tomatoes
1 clove garlic, peeled and crushed
1 small onion, peeled and grated
1 stick celery, grated
1 small carrot, peeled and grated
1 tablespoon soy sauce
1 tablespoon freshly chopped parsley
1 tablespoon fresh lemon juice
2 teaspoons cider vinegar
150–200ml (5–7fl oz) apple juice

method

1 Place all the Barbecue Sauce ingredients in a pan and bring to the boil. Reduce the heat and simmer for about 3–4 minutes to soften the vegetables. Cool slightly and blend in a food processor until smooth. Reheat to serve.

2 For the kebabs, cut the tofu into 12 chunks and thread onto skewers with the vegetables. Brush with a little oil and cook over a barbecue or under a grill for about 5–6 minutes, depending on how seared you like your vegetables.

3 Remove from the grill and serve on a bed of rice. Serve the Barbecue Sauce separately.

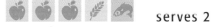 serves 2

grilled sea bass on a bed of swiss chard

Every part of this dish cooks quickly so you need to have everything prepared and ready to go before the start. Cook the Swiss chard first and then the fish. Serve with fresh noodles or tiny new potatoes boiled in their skins.

ingredients

400g (14oz) Swiss chard or spinach, washed and drained
2 fillets sea bass, from a 600g (1lb 5oz) fish
2 teaspoons extra-virgin olive oil
freshly ground black pepper (to taste)
2–3 spring onions, trimmed and roughly sliced
1 level tablespoon toasted pine nuts
a pinch of grated nutmeg

method

1 Steam the Swiss chard or spinach in its own liquid until it is just *al dente*. Drain and keep on one side.

2 Wash the sea bass fillets and dry carefully on kitchen paper. Brush with a very little olive oil and sprinkle with black pepper. Place under a hot grill, flesh side up. Cook for a couple of minutes and turn over so that the skin side faces the heat. Cook for a further 3–4 minutes, depending on the thickness of the fish fillets, until the flesh is cooked through.

3 Place the remaining oil in a heavy-based saucepan and toss the spring onions in it for a minute or so. Roughly chop the Swiss chard or spinach and add to the pan with the pine nuts and nutmeg. Toss together over a medium heat.

4 To assemble the dish, arrange the Swiss chard or spinach on two serving plates and place the grilled sea bass on top.

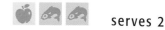 serves 2

sesame grilled chicken on celeriac mash with green beans

The celeriac mash is quite soft and creamy. If you prefer a firmer texture, or are particularly hungry, mash a large cooked potato with the celeriac.

ingredients

2 small chicken breast fillets, skinned
1 tablespoon potato flour
1 small egg, beaten
5–6 tablespoons sesame seeds
150g (5½oz) green beans, trimmed

CELERIAC MASH
400g (14oz) celeriac
2 tablespoons low-fat fromage frais
a little salt
freshly ground black pepper (to taste)

method

1 Cut the chicken fillets into two or three pieces. Coat very lightly with flour, dip in beaten egg and then dip in the sesame seeds. Make sure they are well coated.

2 Place the coated fillets in the grill pan under a hot grill and cook for about 5 minutes on each side until thoroughly cooked. The cut flesh should not show any pink at all.

3 To make the Celeriac Mash, peel and slice the celeriac. Cook in a steamer until tender. Then place in a blender and purée, or mash with a potato masher, and mix with the other ingredients.

4 Cook the green beans in a steamer or in a very little water until they are *al dente* or still slightly crisp to the bite. Serve with the Sesame Grilled Chicken and Celeriac Mash.

serves 2

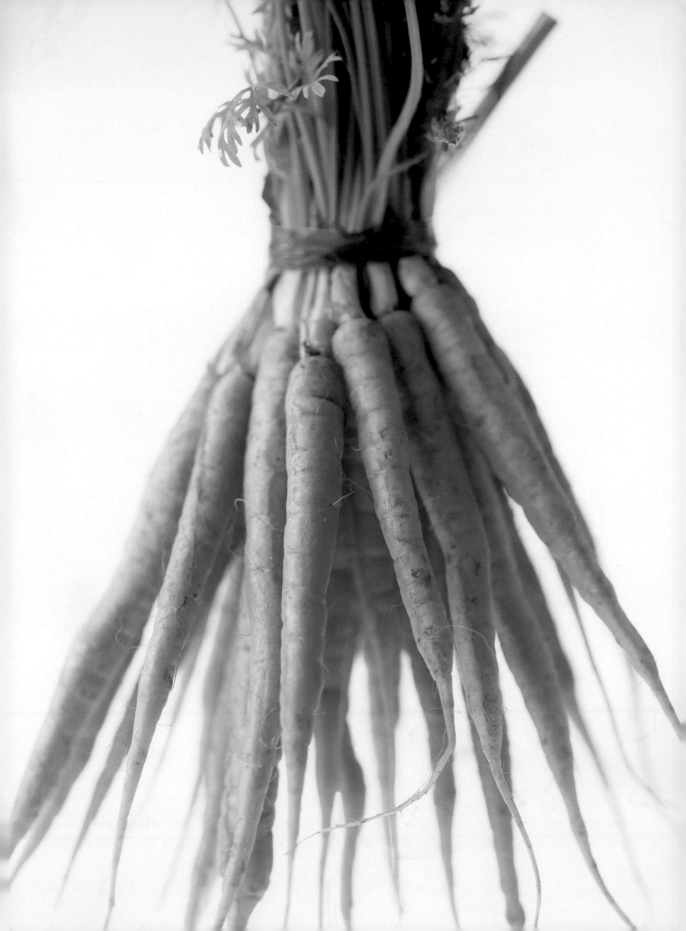

grilled carrot and tofu cakes with red peppers and fennel

You can use any kind of bread to make the breadcrumbs for this recipe but day-old pieces of Tomato Scofa Bread (see page 46) really add to the flavour.

ingredients

2 large red peppers, seeded and cut into large pieces
200g (7oz) firm tofu, mashed with a potato masher
125g (4½oz) carrots, scrubbed and finely grated
50g (2oz) fresh rye or wholemeal breadcrumbs
25g (1oz) ground almonds
4–5 spring onions, trimmed and finely chopped
1 clove garlic, peeled and crushed
1 tablespoon soy sauce
freshly ground black pepper (to taste)
1 tablespoon sesame seeds
1 large head fennel, trimmed and thinly sliced
a few sprigs of fresh parsley

method

1 Prepare the peppers. Then take about a quarter of one pepper and chop very finely, keeping the other pieces on one side.

2 In a large bowl, mix the chopped pepper with the mashed tofu, grated carrots, breadcrumbs, ground almonds, spring onions and garlic. Stir in the soy sauce and black pepper. Then shape the mixture into four cakes and press down so that they are not too thick. Coat each side with a few sesame seeds.

3 Place the Carrot and Tofu Cakes on a piece of foil under a hot grill and add the pieces of red pepper and the sliced fennel. Cook for about 10 minutes on each side until the Carrot and Tofu Cakes are cooked and the vegetables are lightly browned.

4 Arrange the Carrot and Tofu Cakes on two serving plates with the grilled vegetables around them. Garnish with sprigs of fresh parsley.

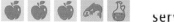 serves 2

flash-grilled tuna in lemon ginger marinade with quinoa and red pepper salsa

The best way to cook tuna is to flash-grill thin slices on a pre-heated ridged grill. This cooks the fish very fast and also leaves attractive markings across it.

ingredients

300g (14oz) fresh tuna, cut into thin slices
cooked quinoa (see page 37)
a little cold-pressed mixed seed oil

MARINADE
juice and grated rind of 1 large or 1½ small lemons
50ml (2fl oz) dry white wine
2 tablespoons soy sauce
1 tablespoon saffron oil *or* ordinary olive oil with a pinch of saffron
6 spring onions, very finely chopped
1 clove garlic, peeled and crushed
1 tablespoon freshly grated ginger

RED PEPPER SALSA
1 red pepper, seeded and finely diced
½ small red chilli pepper, seeded and finely chopped
1 small cucumber, finely diced
2 tablespoons freshly chopped celery or fennel
3 tablespoons freshly chopped coriander
juice of ½ lemon
a little cold-pressed mixed seed oil (optional)

method

1 Place the tuna slices in a shallow non-metallic entrée dish. Mix all the Marinade ingredients together and pour over the fish. Leave to stand for at least an hour, turning from time to time.

2 Cook the quinoa (see page 37) and make the Red Pepper Salsa by simply mixing all the ingredients together in a bowl.

3 Remove the fish from the Marinade and pour the Marinade into a saucepan. Bring to the boil and leave to simmer while you cook the fish. Brush the tuna pieces with mixed seed oil and grill for 1½–2 minutes on each side.

4 Spoon the quinoa onto two serving plates and top with the tuna steaks. Serve with the cooked Marinade spooned over the top and the Salsa on the side.

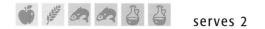 serves 2

salmon tarragon fishcakes with tomato sauce on a bed of spinach

The best way to cook salmon is to poach it for a very short time in a little milk. Remove the fish from the liquid as soon as the flesh turns opaque and you can flake it off the skin or bones. Cook the potatoes in their skins, peel when they are tender and mash.

Ingredients

450g (1lb) salmon, cooked and flaked
225g (8oz) mashed potato
3–4 spring onions, finely chopped
2 tablespoons freshly chopped tarragon
25g (1oz) sesame seeds
25g (1oz) fine breadcrumbs
½ quantity Tomato Sauce (see page 73)
225g (8oz) spinach, washed and drained

method

1 Carefully mix the salmon, potato, spring onions and tarragon, taking care not to break up the flakes of salmon too much.

2 Shape into four large cakes and coat with mixed sesame seeds and breadcrumbs. Place under the grill and cook for about 5 minutes on each side until the fishcakes are browned and heated through.

3 Meanwhile, heat the Tomato Sauce through and gently cook the spinach in its own juices until it just begins to wilt. Drain well and arrange on two serving plates. Place the cooked fishcakes on top. Pour the sauce round the outside of the spinach or over the fishcakes.

 serves 2

lemon and dill turkey escalopes on carrot and tarragon potato mash with beetroot relish

It is much easier to find different cuts of turkey meat these days. Ask your butcher to cut some thin escalopes from the breast and to flatten them for you.

ingredients

zest and juice of ½ lemon
1 tablespoon freshly chopped dill
1 teaspoon extra-virgin olive oil
2 turkey escalopes, well flattened

CARROT AND TARRAGON POTATO MASH
300g (10½ oz) potatoes scrubbed
300g (10½ oz) carrots, peeled and sliced
freshly chopped tarragon (to taste)
1 tablespoon skimmed, soya or rice milk

1 teaspoon extra-virgin olive oil

BEETROOT RELISH
1 medium to large beetroot
zest and juice of ½ lemon
2 spring onions, trimmed and finely chopped
0.5cm (¼ in) thick slice fresh ginger, grated

method

1 Mix the lemon zest and juice with the chopped dill and olive oil and spread over each side of the turkey escalopes. Leave to stand until required to cook.

2 To make the Carrot and Tarragon Potato Mash, steam the potatoes in their skins. Add the carrots to the steamer after about 10 minutes, depending on the size of the potatoes. Cook for another 15–20 minutes until both vegetables are tender.

3 Peel the potatoes and mash with the carrots, tarragon, milk and oil. Beat until smooth.

4 To make the Beetroot Relish, peel the beetroot and shred on the finest part of the grater. Stir in the remaining ingredients and mix well together.

5 Put the escalopes under a hot grill and cook for 2–4 minutes on each side. Check to see that the meat is cooked through. There should be no pinkness in the centre. Serve the escalopes on a bed of Carrot and Tarragon Potato Mash with the Beetroot Relish on the side.

serves 2

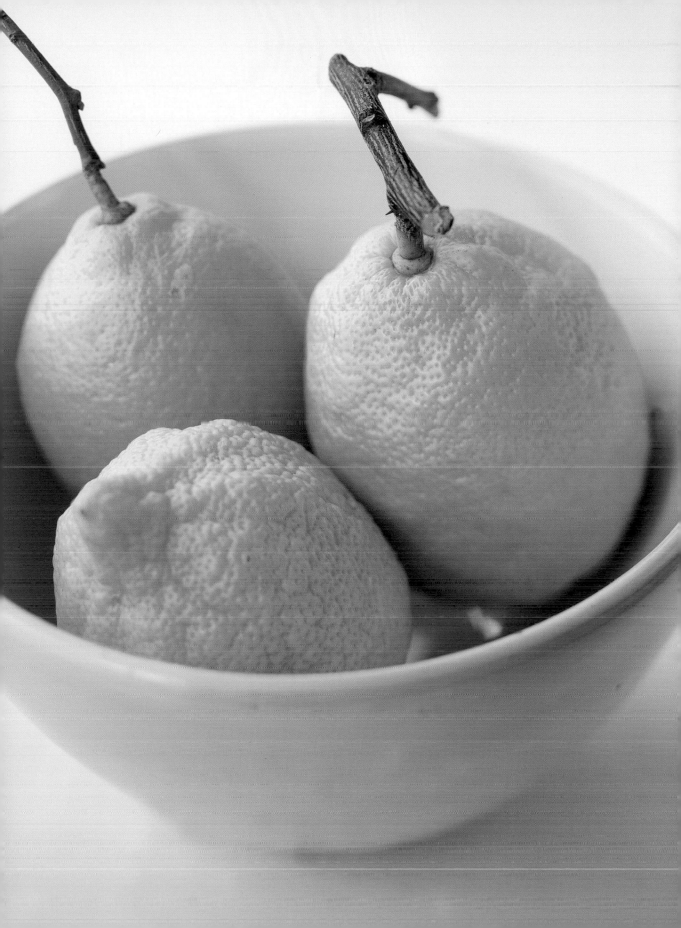

grilled scallops with green sauce, julienne vegetables and rice noodles

This is another recipe where it pays to get all the preparation finished before you start cooking. Begin with the Green Sauce and then prepare the vegetables.

ingredients

2 sticks celery, cut into lengths

100g (3½oz) carrots, peeled and sliced lengthways

100g (3½oz) small French beans, trimmed

1 small red pepper, seeded and sliced

6–8 spring onions, trimmed

50ml (2fl oz) well-flavoured vegetable stock

100–125g (3½–4½oz) rice noodles

12 scallops

a little extra-virgin olive oil

GREEN SAUCE

75g (3oz) spinach, washed and drained

a bunch of chives

25g (1oz) fresh coriander

15g (½oz) fresh basil

1 tablespoon fresh ginger, grated

250ml (9fl oz) well-flavoured vegetable stock

2 tablespoons Greek yoghurt

1–1½ tablespoons potato flour

method

1 To make the Green Sauce, place the spinach in a food processor with the herbs, ginger and stock and blend until smooth. Stir in the yoghurt and pour into a saucepan. Leave to one side until required.

2 Cut all the vegetables into long thin strips and steam-fry in a little stock for 1–2 minutes to soften slightly. Place on one side. Cook the rice noodles as indicated on the pack.

3 Brush the scallops with a little extra-virgin olive oil. Cook under a hot grill for 2½–3 minutes each side until they turn white. Take care not to overcook. If you are not sure, cut one scallop in half – it should be white all the way through.

4 As the scallops are cooking, place the Green Sauce over a medium heat and bring to the boil. Add the potato flour, stirring all the time, until the mixture boils and thickens.

5 Drain the noodles, toss with the steam-fried vegetables and spoon onto two serving plates. Arrange the cooked scallops on the noodles and drizzle the Green Sauce over the top. Alternatively, you could coat the plate with the sauce first.

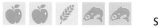 **serves 2**

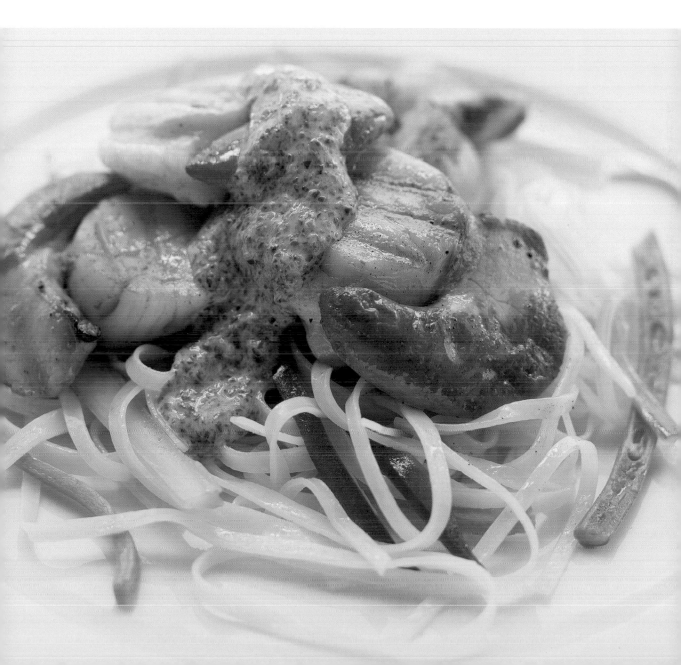

spicy mackerel with couscous

*North Africa provides the inspiration for this spicy sauce but take care with the harissa —
some brands can be very hot indeed. Couscous is the traditional North African carbohydrate
but you could use bulgar or quinoa instead.*

ingredients

a little extra-virgin olive oil
1 small onion, peeled and chopped
1 clove garlic, peeled and crushed
1 teaspoon ground cumin
½–1 teaspoon harissa or chilli powder
1 small red pepper, seeded and chopped
125g (4½oz) courgettes, diced
1 x 200g (7oz) can tomatoes
couscous
1 good-sized mackerel, approximately 300–350g (10½–12 oz), cut into 2 fillets

method

1 Preheat the oven to 180°C/350°F/Gas 4.

2 Heat the oil in a small heavy-based saucepan and stir-fry the onion and garlic with the
cumin and harissa or chilli powder for 1–2 minutes. Add the red pepper and courgettes and
cook for another 2 minutes, stirring all the time.

3 Pour on the tomatoes and bring to the boil. Simmer for 10 minutes, stirring from time to
time. Cook the couscous as directed on the packet.

4 Place the mackerel fillets on a non-stick baking tray and cover with foil. Bake in the oven for
10 minutes or until the fish is cooked through.

5 Arrange the fish on a mound of couscous and top with the sauce.

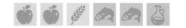

serves 2

minted trout with grapefruit rice salad

It's important to use fresh mint for this recipe. Dried mint simply does not taste the same. Look for good, large fresh sprigs. The same goes for parsley, but it does not really matter whether you choose the curly English variety or the broadleaf Continental type.

ingredients

2 trout, cleaned
a little extra-virgin olive oil
freshly ground black pepper (to taste)
3–4 sprigs fresh mint

GRAPEFRUIT RICE SALAD
100g (3½oz) long-grain rice
200–225ml (7–8fl oz) vegetable stock
1 large grapefruit, peeled
½ green pepper, seeded and very finely chopped
2 tablespoons freshly chopped parsley
1 tablespoon freshly chopped mint

method

1 Start by making the Grapefruit Rice Salad. Place the rice and stock in a saucepan and bring to the boil. Stir and cover. Reduce the heat and cook for 15–18 minutes until all the liquid has been absorbed and the rice is tender.

2 Remove all the pith from the grapefruit and divide it into segments. Chop and trim the segments and remove any pips. Retain the juice that comes out of the fruit as you prepare it. Fluff up the rice with a fork and stir in the prepared grapefruit and its juice. Add all the remaining salad ingredients and mix well. Keep on one side to serve with the trout when it is cooked.

3 Slash the trout across each side twice with a sharp knife. Brush inside and out with olive oil and season with pepper. Put the sprigs of mint in the cavity. Place under a hot grill and cook for 8–10 minutes on each side until the fish is cooked through.

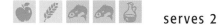

serves 2

top of the stove

thai noodle salad

This colourful vegetable salad, with its warm Thai Dressing, comes from TV chef and author Lesley Waters. She suggests that fish-eaters might like to use 140g (5oz) white crab meat in place of the sugar snap peas and sesame seeds. Serve with Thai Paw (see page 174).

ingredients

100g (3½ oz) thread egg noodles
50g (2oz) sugar snap peas
75g (3oz) spring greens
2 large carrots, peeled
1 tablespoon lightly toasted sesame seeds

DRESSING
2 tablespoons sunflower oil
½ bunch spring onions, cut into chunky strips
1½ tablespoons light soy sauce
juice of ½ large orange
2½ cm (1in) piece fresh root ginger, peeled and grated
1 clove garlic, peeled and crushed
½ teaspoon chopped lemon grass (optional)
1 teaspoon sesame oil
black pepper (to taste)

method

1 Start by making the Dressing. Heat 1 tablespoon of the oil and stir-fry the spring onion for 30 seconds. Remove from the heat and stir in all the remaining Dressing ingredients.

2 To make the Noodle Salad, cook the egg noodles as directed on the pack and drain. Blanch and refresh the peas and spring greens by putting them first in boiling water and then in cold water. Shred the spring greens and cut the peas in half lengthways. Cut the carrots into sticks.

3 Place all the prepared ingredients in a salad bowl and pour on the warm Dressing. Sprinkle with the sesame seeds and serve.

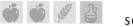

serves 2

chestnut hot pot with beansprout salad

Chestnuts are the lowest-fat nuts by a long way. Fresh chestnuts are on sale in the autumn, and when they are out of season you can buy dried chestnuts or cooked vacuum-packed chestnuts, both of which are much easier to deal with.

ingredients

100g (3½oz) dried chestnuts or 200g (7oz) cooked chestnuts
1 medium onion, peeled and sliced
2 cloves garlic, peeled and crushed
1 teaspoon extra-virgin olive oil
200ml (7fl oz) vegetable stock
150g (5½oz) carrots, peeled and sliced
125g (4½oz) turnip, peeled and sliced
1 x 200g (7oz) can tomatoes
freshly ground black pepper (to taste)
a pinch of dried thyme

BEANSPROUT SALAD
150g (5½oz) mung bean sprouts or mixed beansprouts
½ red or green pepper, seeded and sliced
2 spring onions, finely chopped
juice of ½ lemon

method

1 If using dried chestnuts, soak them overnight and drain well.

2 Place the onion, garlic and oil in a large pan and steam-fry, using a little stock as required, for a couple of minutes. Add the sliced vegetables and cook for a further minute before adding the rest of the stock, the chestnuts, the canned tomatoes, black pepper and thyme.

3 Bring the mixture to the boil, then cover and simmer for 25–30 minutes, stirring occasionally, until the vegetables are cooked. (You may need longer if you are using dried chestnuts.)

4 Place all the Beansprout Salad ingredients in a large bowl and toss well together. Serve with the Hot Pot.

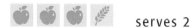

serves 2

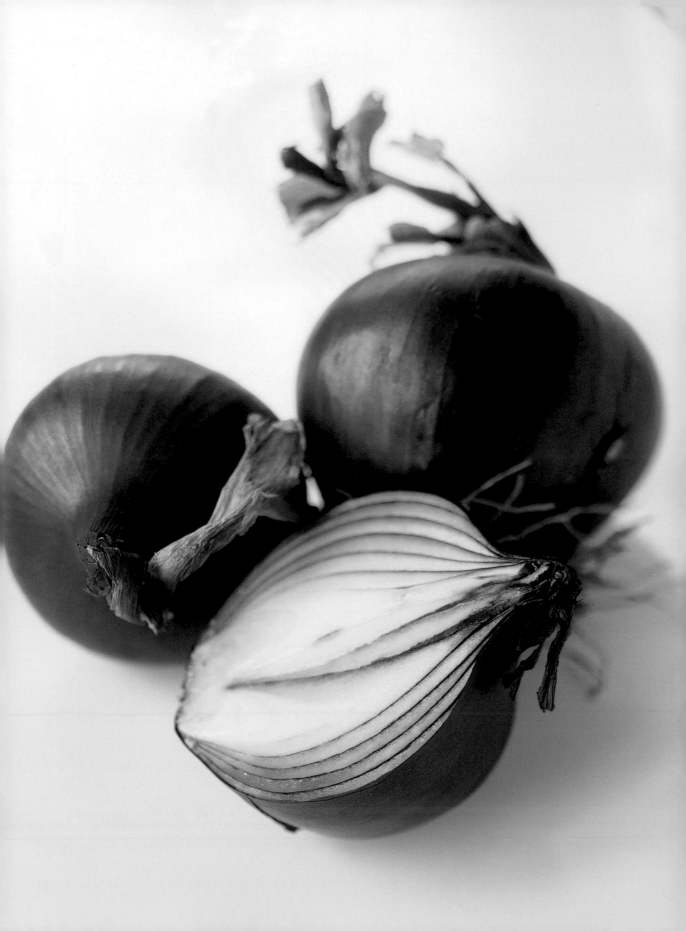

warm avocado, arame, rice and quinoa salad with rainbow roots

This salad is good warm but it can also be served cold later in the day.

ingredients

SALAD
50g (2oz) rice
25g (1oz) quinoa
3 shallots or 1 small onion, peeled and sliced
1 clove garlic, peeled and crushed
1 dessertspoon extra-virgin olive oil
40g (1½oz) sun-dried peppers, soaked in boiling water
25g (1oz) arame, soaked in cold water
1 large avocado, peeled and sliced
2 spring onions, finely chopped
2 tablespoons lemon juice

RAINBOW ROOTS
2 medium carrots, peeled and coarsely grated
½ small celeriac or a small parsnip, peeled and grated
1 small beetroot, grated
1 tablespoon extra-virgin olive oil
1 teaspoon lemon juice or cider vinegar

method

1 To make the Salad, cook the rice with the quinoa in 175–200ml (6½–8fl oz) water for about 15–20 minutes until both are tender. In another pan, cook shallots or the onion and garlic in the olive oil for a minute or two to soften. Place the cooked rice in a bowl and stir in the onion and garlic.

2 Drain the peppers and arame and dry on kitchen paper. Add to the rice mixture with all the remaining Salad ingredients and toss well together.

3 Combine all the Rainbow Roots ingredients and toss well together. Serve with the Salad.

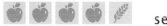

serves 2

teriyaki salmon with tossed steam-fry vegetable noodles

You can choose any kind of noodles for this recipe.

ingredients

2 fresh salmon fillets, approximately 150–175g (5½–6oz) each
1 heaped tablespoon freshly grated root ginger
2 spring onions
2 tablespoons teriyaki or soy sauce
2 tablespoons sherry, white wine or water
some fresh herbs (e.g. parsley, chervil or dill)

TOSSED STEAM-FRY VEGETABLE NOODLES
2 sticks celery
1 small red pepper, seeded
16–20 mangetout
6–8 spring onions
1 teaspoon extra-virgin olive oil
100–150g (3½–5½oz) noodles

method

1 To make the Steam-Fry Vegetable Noodles, put a large pan of water on to boil.

2 Cut the vegetables into thin sticks, then steam-fry in the olive oil and a little water for about 3 minutes until cooked to your liking.

3 Add the noodles to the boiling water and cook for about 3 minutes or as directed on the pack. Drain and add to the vegetables.

4 Place the salmon fillets, skin side down, on two serving plates and spread with grated ginger. Finely chop two of the spring onions and sprinkle over the fillets with the teriyaki or soy sauce and the sherry, white wine or water.

5 Fill two large saucepans with water and bring to the boil. Reduce the heat and place one plate on each pan. Cover the salmon fillets with another plate, and leave to steam for about 7 minutes. Very carefully turn the fillets over and steam for a further 5–7 minutes, depending on the thickness of the salmon, until the fish is cooked through. Take care not to over-cook. Drain the juice into the Steam-Fry Vegetable Noodles.

6 Pile the noodles onto two serving plates. Very carefully arrange the salmon fillets on top. Garnish with fresh herbs and serve.

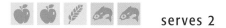 serves 2

vegetarian chilli with taco shells and green salad

It's fun to serve this Vegetarian Chilli in taco shells. Serve with a green salad.

ingredients

1 small onion, peeled and finely chopped

1 clove garlic, peeled and crushed

1 teaspoon extra-virgin olive oil

125g (4½ oz) mushrooms, finely chopped

1 small aubergine, finely diced

1 tablespoon tomato purée

100ml (3½ fl oz) vegetable stock

1–2 teaspoons chilli powder (to taste)

½ teaspoon ground cumin

a pinch of mixed dried herbs

150g (5½ oz) red kidney beans, cooked or canned and drained

6–8 taco shells

method

1 Gently cook the onion and garlic in the olive oil until soft. Add the mushrooms, aubergines, tomato purée, stock, spices and herbs and bring to the boil.

2 Reduce the heat and simmer for 30 minutes, stirring from time to time. Stir in the kidney beans and cook for a further 10 minutes.

3 Heat the taco shells (as directed on the pack), stuff with the chilli mixture and serve.

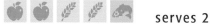 serves 2

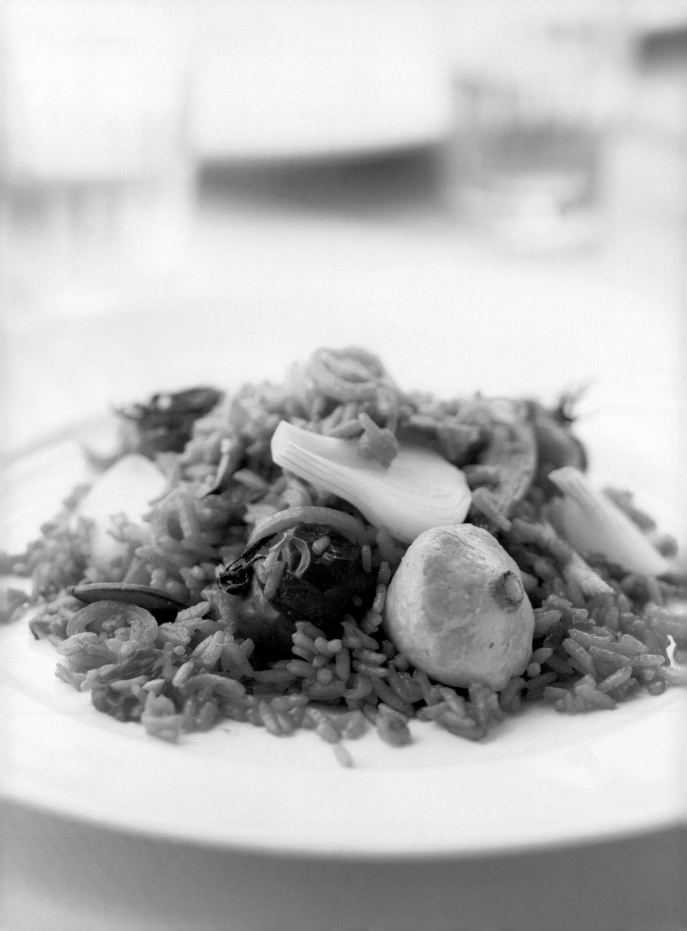

garden paella

This recipe can be made with the vegetables alone but, if you like, you could add a small quantity of cooked chicken, shellfish or marinated tofu at the end of cooking.

ingredients

2 shallots or 1 small onion, peeled and finely chopped
2 cloves garlic, peeled and chopped
1 teaspoon extra-virgin olive oil
1 very ripe beef tomato, skinned, seeded and chopped
¼ teaspoon powdered saffron
a pinch of cayenne pepper
175g (6oz) risotto or long-grain rice
8 bulbous spring onions
8–10 baby sweetcorn
400ml (14fl oz) good vegetable stock
75g (3oz) green beans
6–8 baby courgettes or patty pan squashes
75g (3oz) sugar snap peas
6–8 cherry tomatoes

method

1 Gently cook the shallots or onion and garlic in the olive oil until they begin to soften. Next, add the chopped tomato and cook quickly until all the liquid has evaporated.

2 Add the saffron, cayenne pepper and rice to the tomato mixture and stir well so that all the rice is coated.

3 Place the spring onions and baby sweetcorn on top of the rice and pour on the stock. Cook over a low heat for 10 minutes.

4 Add the beans, courgettes or squashes and sugar snap peas and cook for 10 more minutes.

5 Finally, add the cherry tomatoes and heat through for about 5 minutes. Serve from the pan.

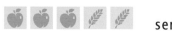 **serves 2**

mushroom stroganoff with rice and quinoa pilaf

Here's a wonderfully aromatic alternative to Beef Stroganoff. Serve with a good pilaf – this one is made with rice and quinoa – and a green salad.

ingredients

15g (½ oz) dried porcini mushrooms
1 onion, peeled and chopped
1 tablespoon extra-virgin olive oil
100g (3½ oz) shiitake mushrooms, halved or quartered
100g (3½ oz) closed-cup mushrooms, halved or quartered
2 cloves garlic, peeled and crushed
1 fresh red chilli, seeded and chopped
1 large tomato, skinned and chopped
1 teaspoon potato flour
50g (2oz) Greek yoghurt
1 tablespoon freshly chopped coriander

RICE AND QUINOA PILAF
1 teaspoon extra-virgin olive oil
1 small onion, trimmed, peeled and finely chopped
70g (3oz) long-grain rice
50g (2oz) quinoa
3 tablespoons frozen peas
275–300ml (10–11fl oz) water or vegetable stock
freshly ground black pepper (to taste)

method

1 Soak the porcini mushrooms in 50ml (2fl oz) boiling water for 10–15 minutes. Gently sweat the onion in the oil for 2–3 minutes to soften. Add the remaining mushrooms and steam-fry with the juices from the dried porcini.

2 After about 5 minutes add the garlic, chilli and tomato and a further 150ml (5fl oz) water or vegetable stock. Bring to the boil. Reduce the heat and simmer for 10 minutes.

3 Meanwhile, to make the Pilaf, heat the oil in a heavy-based pan and gently fry the onion.

Add the rice, quinoa and peas, and stir well. Pour on the water or stock and season with black pepper.

4 Bring to the boil, reduce the heat, cover and simmer for 15–20 minutes until the grains are tender and all the liquid has been absorbed. Fluff up with a fork and serve at once with the Mushroom Stroganoff.

5 Make a creamy paste with the potato flour and a little water and stir into the Stroganoff with the yoghurt. Add the fresh coriander and return to the boil. As soon as the mixture thickens, serve with the Pilaf.

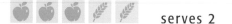 **serves 2**

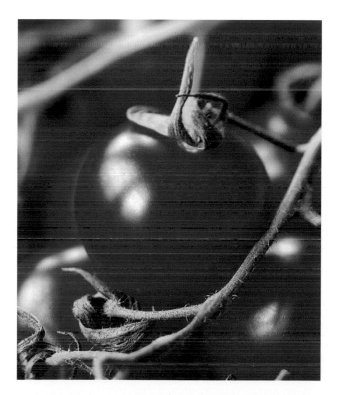

giambotta with mixed green vegetables

This luscious vegetable casserole comes from Ursula Ferrigno, author of Real Fast Vegetarian Food.

ingredients

GIAMBOTTA
1 tablespoon extra-virgin olive oil
1 medium onion, peeled and chopped
1 clove garlic, peeled and crushed
1 small aubergine, trimmed and cut into cubes
1 large red pepper, seeded and cut into chunks
1 courgette, trimmed and sliced
2 potatoes, peeled and cut into cubes
2 teaspoons fennel seeds, crushed
400g (14oz) can tomatoes
6 tablespoons red wine
salt and pepper (to taste)

MIXED GREEN VEGETABLES
100g (3½ oz) French beans, trimmed
100g (3½ oz) runner beans, trimmed and sliced
100g (3½ oz) sugar snap peas, trimmed

method

1 For the Giambotta, heat the oil in a heavy-based saucepan and add the onions and garlic. Cook for about 3–4 minutes to brown them lightly.

2 Add all the remaining Giambotta ingredients and bring to the boil. Cover with a lid, reduce the heat and simmer for 30 minutes or until the potatoes are cooked through.

3 Remove the lid, turn up the heat and cook until the liquid reduces and the mixture thickens.

4 For the Mixed Green Vegetables, place all the beans and peas in the top of a steamer with boiling water in the base. Steam for about 6–8 minutes until the vegetables are just cooked but still slightly crunchy. Serve with the Giambotta.

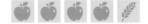 serves 2

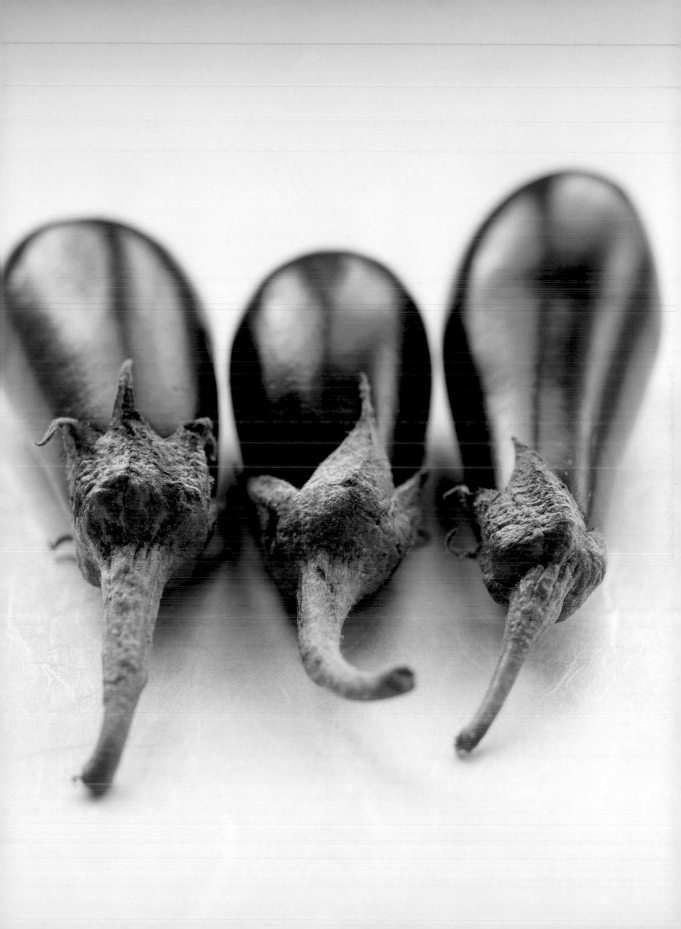

indian vegan feast with okra in curried tomato sauce, gujerati spiced cabbage, tarka dhal and southern indian coconut rice

This is an unashamed mixture of culinary ideas from a range of Indian cuisines but they all work well together. Beware the fat content if you are watching your weight or your heart. We have tried to keep the fat to a minimum but the flavours depend on some traditional frying. The quantities serve four people.

ingredients

OKRA IN CURRIED TOMATO SAUCE
450g (1lb) small okra
2 onions, peeled and sliced
2 cloves garlic, peeled and chopped
2 teaspoons olive oil
2 teaspoons garam masala or medium curry powder
2 teaspoons ground cumin
2 teaspoons ground turmeric
1 teaspoon ground coriander
8 tomatoes, skinned and chopped
freshly ground black pepper (to taste)
juice of 1 lemon

GUJERATI SPICED CABBAGE
1 tablespoon sunflower or corn oil
$\frac{1}{2}$ teaspoon whole cumin seeds
1 onion, peeled and sliced
175g (6oz) green cabbage, very finely shredded
100g (3$\frac{1}{2}$oz) curly kale, very finely shredded
100g (3$\frac{1}{2}$oz) carrots, peeled and coarsely grated
1 small fresh green chilli, shredded and cut into very thin strips
4 tablespoons vegetable stock or water
2 heaped tablespoons freshly chopped coriander
1 tablespoon lemon juice

TARKA DHAL

175g (6oz) split lentils, washed and picked over

1 teaspoon turmeric

2 tablespoons vegetable oil

1–3 dried chillies

1 teaspoon whole cumin seeds

1 small onion, peeled and thinly sliced

1 clove garlic, peeled and crushed

salt and freshly ground black pepper (to taste)

SOUTHERN INDIAN COCONUT RICE

150g (5½ oz) long-grain rice

300–325ml (10–11fl oz) coconut milk

2 whole cardamom pods

1 stick cinnamon

6 black peppercorns

a pinch of sugar

50g (2oz) desiccated coconut

method **1** To make the Okra, cut the stems away, taking care not to cut into the main body of the vegetable.

2 Fry the onions and garlic in the olive oil until very lightly browned. Stir in the ground spices, chopped tomatoes and pepper. Cook for a couple of minutes to soften the tomatoes.

3 Add the okra and toss the ingredients together. Bring to the boil, cover and simmer for about 10–15 minutes until the okra is tender. Take care not to overcook the okra or it will go mushy and slimy. Just before serving, pour on the lemon juice and toss the okra well.

4 For the Gujerati Spiced Cabbage, heat the oil in a frying pan and fry the cumin seeds until they begin to pop. Quickly add the onion and then the cabbage, kale, carrots and green chilli and turn the heat down to medium.

5 Stir-fry the vegetables for 3–4 minutes. Add the stock or water and cook for a further 3–4 minutes, covered with a lid. Stir from time to time. Just before serving, add the chopped coriander, pour on the lemon juice and toss the vegetables well.

6 To make the Tarka Dhal, put the lentils into a pan with 700ml (23fl oz) water and the turmeric and bring to the boil. Cover and simmer for 40–45 minutes, stirring occasionally.

7 Heat the vegetable oil in a small frying pan and fry the whole chillies and cumin seeds for about a minute. Add the onion and garlic to the pan and continue frying briskly until the onion is well browned. Stir this mixture into the cooked lentils and season with a little salt and black pepper.

8 For the Southern Indian Coconut Rice, place the rice in a saucepan with the coconut milk, the whole spices and the sugar. Bring to the boil, stir and cover with a lid. Cook over a low heat for 15–20 minutes depending on the type of rice you are using.

9 Toast the desiccated coconut on a piece of foil under the grill, taking care not to burn it. When the rice is cooked fluff up with a fork and serve with the toasted coconut sprinkled over the top.

serves 4

egg pilau with celeriac and salsa de mojo

Salsa de Mojo is another fragrant recipe from Ursula Ferrigno (author of Real Fast Vegetarian Food*). She uses this piquant sauce, unique to the Canary Islands, on boiled potatoes and seasonal vegetables but her favourite combination is with celeriac.*

Here we have added a delicate Egg Pilau which also goes well with the sauce but you can easily substitute new potatoes if you are in a hurry or cannot tolerate eggs.

ingredients

EGG PILAU
a pinch of whole cumin seeds
1 teaspoon extra-virgin olive oil
a pinch of dried thyme
1 small onion, peeled and finely chopped
½ teaspoon ground turmeric
125g (4½ oz) long-grain rice
2 hard-boiled eggs, roughly chopped

SALSA DE MOJO

1–2 cloves garlic (to taste)

$^1/_2$ teaspoon cumin seeds

$^1/_2$ teaspoon paprika

1$^1/_2$–2 teaspoons fresh thyme leaves

25ml (1fl oz) extra-virgin olive oil

1 teaspoon wine vinegar

500g (1lb 2oz) celeriac

method

1 To make the Egg Pilau, quickly fry the cumin in the oil, add the thyme and onion and continue frying for one minute. Add the turmeric and rice and 250–275ml (9–9$^1/_2$fl oz) water, and bring to the boil. Stir once and cover with a lid. Cook over a low heat for 15–20 minutes, depending on the type of rice you are using.

2 For the Salsa, peel the garlic and crush in a mortar with the cumin seeds. Grind until fine. Add the paprika and thyme and add the olive oil a drop at a time until well mixed. Add the vinegar and then 25ml (1fl oz) water and leave to cool. Peel and slice the celeriac and cook in a steamer until tender.

3 When the rice is cooked, fluff it up with a fork and stir in the chopped eggs. Serve with the celeriac and Salsa de Mojo.

serves 2

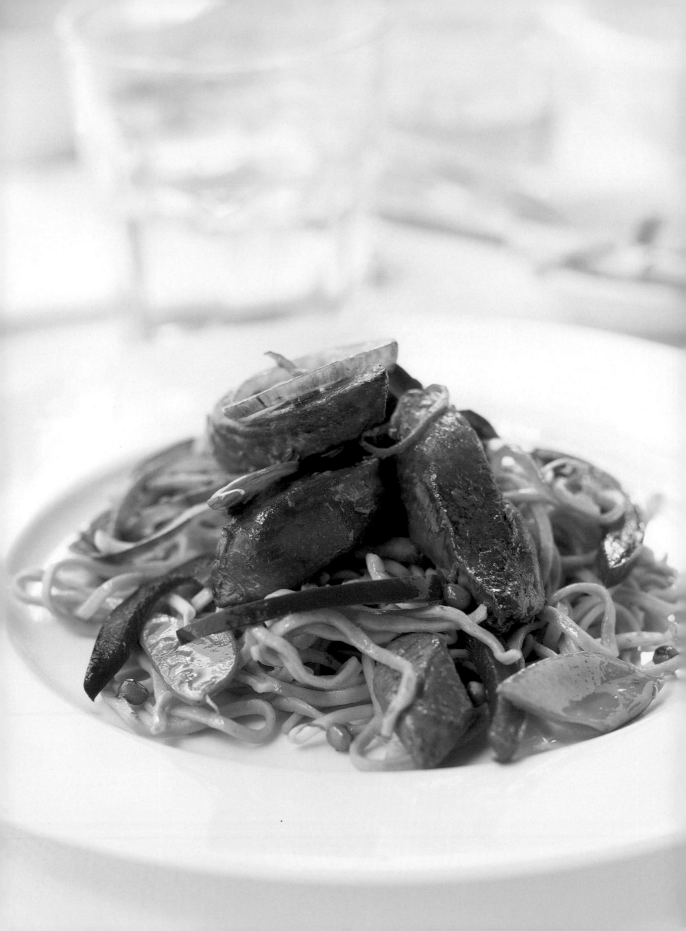

duck slivers with orange beansprouts and chinese egg noodles

This is another 'East meets West' dish – a Chinese treatment of the Western combination of duck and orange. The very best duck to use is wild duck or mallard, as these birds have very little fat. Failing that, use a large Barbary duck breast and remove all the fatty skin.

ingredients

1 onion, peeled and sliced

2 cloves garlic, peeled and chopped

0.5cm (¼in) thick slice of fresh root ginger, peeled and cut into thin sticks

1 teaspoon extra-virgin olive oil

about 2 tablespoons soy sauce

2 mallard breasts or 1 barbary duck breast, skinned and cut into strips

juice and zest of ½ orange

1 small red pepper, seeded and cut into strips

100g (3½ oz) mangetout

a pinch of five-spice powder

150g (5½ oz) mung beansprouts

Chinese egg noodles (to serve 2)

method

1 Steam-fry the onion, garlic and ginger in the olive oil and a little soy sauce. Add the duck slivers and continue to steam-fry for about 5 minutes until the duck is cooked through. Remove from the pan and keep warm.

2 Cut the orange zest into very thin slivers and steam-fry with the red pepper and a little more soy sauce. Add the mangetout, orange juice and five spice powder and cook for a further minute or so. Add the beansprouts and toss well together. Mix in the reserved duck and any juices.

3 Meanwhile, cook the egg noodles as directed on the pack and then serve straight away with the duck.

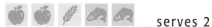

serves 2

thai green curry with fragrant rice and thai paw

This is a very traditional Thai curry made with green curry paste. Vary the amount of paste to suit the level of heat you prefer in the dish.

The recipe for Thai Paw comes from Lesley Waters' book Broader than Beans. *She suggests also trying it as a starter or as a cooler after a really hot curry. Take care, though: it has plenty of its own chilli heat.*

ingredients

THAI GREEN CURRY
1 onion, peeled and chopped
2 cloves garlic, peeled and crushed
2 heaped teaspoons green curry paste
1 teaspoon extra-virgin olive oil
1 dessertspoon fish sauce
1 large chicken breast fillet, skinned and cut into chunks
or 250g (9oz) firm tofu, cut into cubes
1 x 400ml (14fl oz) can coconut milk
2 kaffir lime leaves or a large piece of dried galangal
100g (3½ oz) Thai fragrant rice
1 large courgette, approximately 200g (7oz), cut into slices
a handful of fresh basil or coriander leaves

THAI PAW
juice of 1 lime
1 fresh red chilli, seeded and finely chopped
2 spring onions, sliced diagonally
1 large, just-ripe paw-paw (also known as papaya) or mango
salt and black pepper (to taste)
a handful of fresh coriander leaves
lime wedges (to serve)

method **1** Steam-fry the onion, garlic and curry paste in the oil for 2 minutes. Add the fish sauce, chicken and tofu and continue to cook for another 2–3 minutes.

2 Add the coconut milk and kaffir lime leaves or galangal. Bring the mixture to the boil. Stir, cover and simmer for at least an hour.

3 About 15 minutes before serving, place the rice and 200ml (7fl oz) water in a saucepan and bring to the boil. Stir, cover and simmer for about 12 minutes until the rice is cooked through. Leave to stand for 1–2 minutes.

4 About 5 minutes before serving, add the courgette and basil or coriander leaves to the chicken curry.

5 To make the Thai Paw, combine the lime juice, chilli and spring onion in a small bowl. Quarter the paw-paw (or mango) and scoop out the seeds (or remove the stone). Cut off the skin and cut the flesh into small chunks. Add to the lime and chilli mixture and season. Gently stir in the coriander leaves and serve with the lime wedges.

6 Serve the chicken curry with the Thai fragrant rice and Thai Paw.

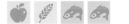 **serves 2**

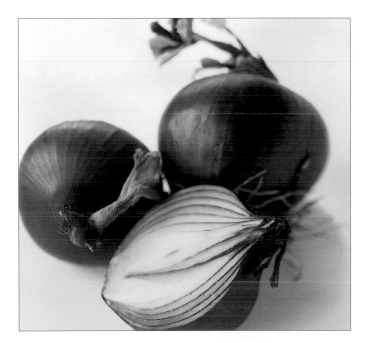

oriental seafood with sushi rice

Serve this dish with pickled ginger which you can buy at Oriental delicatessen shops.

ingredients

250ml (9fl oz) stock or water

1 tablespoon tamari or soy sauce

0.5cm (¼in) thick slice fresh root ginger, peeled and cut into thin strips

1 small onion, peeled and sliced

15g (½oz) dried arame seaweed, soaked in cold water

125g (4½oz) mangetout, trimmed

200g (7oz) pak choy, coarsely chopped

75g (3oz) King prawns

1 small lemon sole or plaice, filleted, skinned and cut into large pieces

4 spring onions, trimmed and diagonally sliced

SUSHI RICE

125g (4½oz) long-grain rice   1 teaspoon sugar

2 tablespoons rice vinegar or cider vinegar   salt (to taste)

method

1 For the Sushi Rice, soak the rice in cold water for an hour before cooking. Drain and place in a pan with 150ml (5fl oz) water. Bring to the boil. Stir, cover and simmer for 12 minutes. meanwhile mix the vinegar with the sugar and salt and heat through in a small pan.

2 To cook the fish, place the stock or water in a large saucepan and add the tamari or soy sauce, ginger and onion and bring to the boil. Simmer for 10 minutes. Add the arame, mangetout and pak choy and cook for a further 5 minutes.

3 Add the prawns, stir and arrange the pieces of fish on the top. Turn up the heat. Cover and cook for about 3 minutes until the fish has turned opaque and is cooked through. Sprinkle with the chopped spring onion.

4 Turn the cooked fish into a bowl. Pour the vinegar mixture equally all over the rice and stir in with a fork. Serve the fish with the rice on the side with some ginger pickle arranged on top.

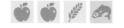 serves 2

baked in the oven

mexican spinach with baked yams

The inspiration for this dish comes from South America.

ingredients

2 small yams
700g (1lb 9oz) spinach
1 green pepper
1 onion, peeled and finely chopped
2–3 sticks celery, finely chopped
1 teaspoon extra-virgin olive oil
½ teaspoon ground cinnamon
a pinch of cayenne pepper
a pinch of dill or fennel seeds
50ml (2fl oz) tomato juice
salt and pepper (to taste)
25g (1oz) raisins
50g (2oz) grated Cheddar cheese

method

1 Preheat the oven to 190°C/375°F/Gas 5.

2 Cut the yams in half lengthways and place on a baking tray. Bake for 60–90 minutes, depending on the thickness of the yams.

3 Wash the spinach and drain well. Cook in a large pan for 5 minutes until it wilts. Seed and slice the green pepper and blanch for 5 minutes in boiling water. Steam-fry the onion and celery in the olive oil with the spices and seeds, adding the tomato juice as you go.

4 Place half the spinach in the base of a large oval earthenware dish. Add a layer of peppers and then all of the onion and celery mix. Sprinkle with the raisins and half the cheese. Cover with the remaining peppers and then the spinach. Finish off with the last of the cheese and season as required. Bake for 45 minutes and serve with the yams.

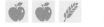

serves 2

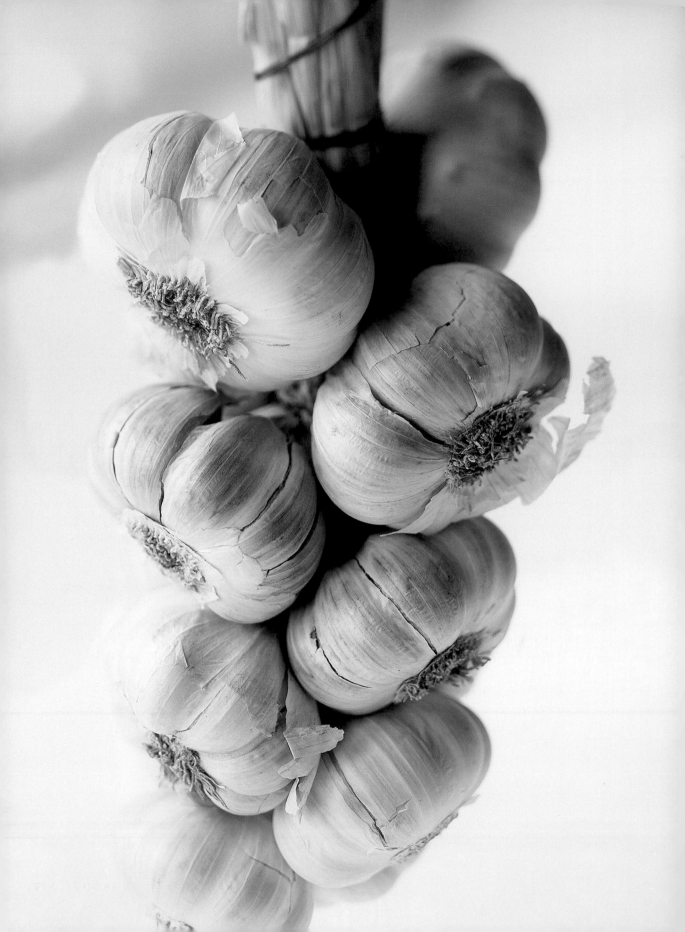

roasted red peppers with goat's cheese and sweet potato mash

Red is the predominant colour in this great match of flavours so I usually add a flash of green in the form of a chopped parsley and rocket salad.

ingredients

2 large red peppers, halved and seeded
1 large clove of garlic, peeled and thinly sliced
2 tomatoes, halved
freshly ground black pepper (to taste)
4–5cm (1½–2in) thick piece Chevre log, approx 200g (7oz), cut into 4 slices
a pinch of dried thyme

SWEET POTATO MASH
2 medium to large sweet potatoes, approximately 400–450g (14–16oz)
2 level tablespoons Greek yoghurt
freshly ground black pepper (to taste)

method

1 Set the oven to 200°C/400°F/Gas 6.

2 Place the red pepper halves in a heatproof dish open side down. Bake in the oven for half an hour.

3 Turn the peppers over, put a few slivers of garlic in the base of each one and fill with half a tomato. Sprinkle with black pepper and return to the oven for a further 15 minutes.

4 Top each pepper half with a slice of goat's cheese and sprinkle with the dried thyme. Bake for another 5–8 minutes until the cheese just begins to run.

5 For the Sweet Potato Mash, place the potatoes in the oven with the peppers and bake for about an hour until they are cooked through. Split open the skins and scoop out the flesh. Mix with the Greek yoghurt and black pepper and serve with the Roasted Red Peppers.

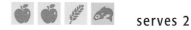 serves 2

pot-roasted guinea fowl with spicy potatoes and wild mushrooms in sesame sauce

This is a good dish for a celebration. Guinea fowl has a more interesting flavour than chicken and it takes well to this simple method of roasting with all its own juices.

The wild mushrooms add a touch of luxury to the meal but if you don't want to spend quite so much you can use small closed-cap mushrooms with about 15g (½oz) dried porcini, or wild mushrooms, soaked in a little boiling water, to pep up the flavour.

ingredients

1 lean guinea fowl, with as much fat as possible removed

2 tablespoons white wine

2 tablespoons vegetable stock

freshly ground black pepper (to taste)

a few sprigs of watercress

SPICY POTATOES

4 large baking potatoes

2 tablespoons extra-virgin olive oil

freshly ground black pepper (to taste)

a few drops of Tabasco sauce

WILD MUSHROOMS IN SESAME SAUCE

2 tablespoons tahini paste

50ml (2fl oz) soya milk

freshly ground black pepper (to taste)

2 large or 4 small shallots, peeled and chopped

1½ tablespoons extra-virgin olive oil

250g (9oz) wild mushrooms (e.g. chanterelles, girolles, ceps and
   trompettes des morts)

1 tablespoon lemon juice

3–4 tablespoons vegetable stock

some chopped fresh parsley

method **1** Set the oven to 200°C/400°F/Gas 6.

2 Place the guinea fowl in a heavy casserole dish and pour on the wine and stock. Add the black pepper and cover with a lid. Place in the oven and roast for an hour until the juices run clear when the guinea fowl is prodded with a fork.

3 Carve the guinea fowl and serve garnished with watercress. Pour the juices from the casserole into a gravy boat to serve as a sauce.

4 The Spicy Potatoes are roasted at the same time and same tempertaure as the Guinea Fowl.

5 Cut the potatoes into 2.5cm (1in) cubes with their skins on. Toss in the olive oil with the pepper and Tabasco and place in a roasting tin. Roast for about an hour, turning the potatoes once or twice.

6 To make the Wild Mushrooms in Sesame Sauce, start by mixing the tahini paste with the soya milk and black pepper in a small saucepan. Place over a low heat and slowly bring to the boil, stirring regularly. The mixture will gradually thicken. Do not cook for too long or the sauce will be too thick.

7 Meanwhile, cook the shallots in the oil for 1–2 minutes and add the mushrooms, lemon juice and stock. Cook for a further minute or two, turning the mushrooms occasionally.

8 Now add the tahini sauce, toss well together, sprinkle with chopped parsley and serve with the Pot-Roasted Guinea Fowl.

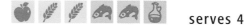 **serves 4**

thai baked fish with steam-fried vegetables

This is a great way to cook almost any kind of fish.

ingredients

2 fish steaks or fillets
1 large clove garlic, peeled and thinly sliced
1 stick lemon grass, cut into two or three pieces
1 red chilli, seeded and thinly sliced
juice and grated zest of 1 lime
1cm (½ in) fresh root ginger, grated
1 tablespoon sesame oil
1 tablespoon soy sauce

STEAM-FRIED VEGETABLES
1 stick celery, sliced
½ green pepper, seeded and sliced
8–10 baby sweetcorn
50ml (2fl oz) vegetable stock
1 leek, trimmed and sliced
100g (3½ oz) mangetout
1 tablespoon soy sauce
50g (2oz) beansprouts
a few sprigs of fresh coriander

method

1 Wash the fish and place in an ovenproof dish. Arrange the garlic, lemon grass and chilli over the top of the fish. Mix all the other ingredients in a cup and pour over the fish. If possible, leave the fish to marinate for an hour. However, this is not essential.

2 Preheat the oven to 190°C/375°F/Gas 5. Cover the fish with foil and bake for 15–30 minutes, depending on the thickness of the fish.

3 For the Steam-Fried Vegetables, steam-fry the celery, pepper and sweetcorn in half the stock. After a few minutes, add the leek and mangetout and the rest of the stock. Continue cooking until the vegetables are cooked the way you like them. Finally, add the soy sauce and beansprouts. Toss well and serve with the fish. Garnish with the sprigs of fresh coriander.

 serves 2

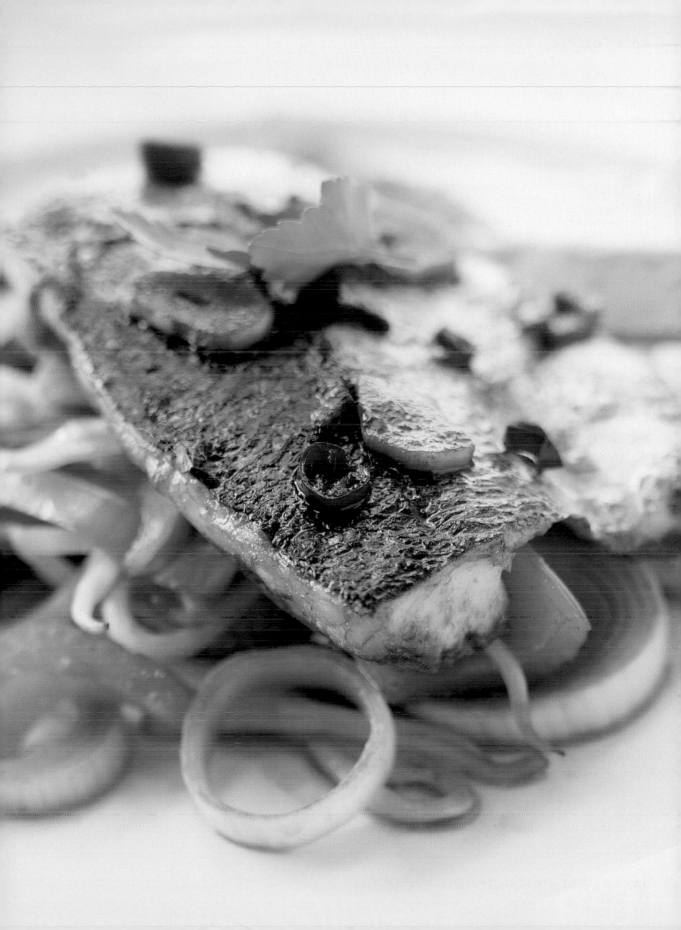

jacket baked potatoes with broccoli and fennel salad

A baked potato is a great base for a satisfying meal. Choose general-purpose or floury varieties such as Marfona, Maris Piper or King Edward, or try sweet potatoes for a change. All potatoes need to be well scrubbed and slit along one side with a sharp knife. Remove any nasty-looking eyes or holes.

You can bake potatoes in a microwave oven but I much prefer them baked in a conventional oven. This is because I like to have really crisp skins and this is impossible to achieve in the microwave. Of course, it is probably healthier to cut the cooking time and eat the potatoes when they are cooked but still firm inside! The choice is yours.

Choose one of these two quite different toppings and serve with the Broccoli and Fennel Salad.

Fresh herbs are the secret of success with the Tofu Topping. If you cannot find the herbs you want in winter, try the new freshly-frozen herbs which are now available in supermarkets.

The Mediterranean Topping is not only good for jacket potatoes. Try it spread on pizza bases and topped with Mozzarella, or served on thin pasta such as spaghettini or linguine.

tofu topping

ingredients

200g (7oz) silken tofu
3–4 tablespoons soya milk
1 tablespoon cold-pressed mixed seed oil
juice of ½ lemon
4–5 large sprigs mixed fresh herbs (e.g. basil, parsley and oregano or mixed parsley and mint)
freshly ground black pepper (to taste)

mediterranean topping

ingredients

2 tomatoes

4 sun-dried tomatoes

1 medium leek

1 courgette

2 large sweet peppers, red and yellow

1 clove garlic

1 teaspoon tomato purée

1 teaspoon extra-virgin olive oil

1 teaspoon cider vinegar

freshly ground black pepper (to taste)

1 fresh red chilli, finely chopped (optional)

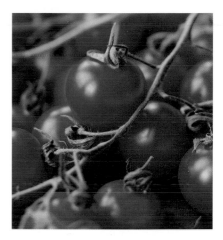

broccoli and fennel salad

ingredients

½ small bulb fennel, chopped

a small head of broccoli, chopped

7cm (3 in) length of cucumber, diced

2 sticks celery, chopped

½ small lettuce

1 tablespoon extra-virgin olive oil

1 teaspoon lemon juice

method

1 Place all the Tofu Topping ingredients in a blender and process until smooth and creamy.

2 For the Mediterranean Topping, seed the tomatoes and cut the sun-dried tomatoes and all the vegetables into small, thin strips. Place in a pan with all the remaining ingredients. Put the pan on a low to medium heat and bring to the boil gradually, stirring from time to time. Cover and simmer for 45 minutes until all the liquid has gone. Stir from time to time.

3 For the Broccoli and Fennel Salad, mix the fennel, broccoli, cucumber and celery in a bowl. Arrange the lettuce leaves on two side plates and spoon on the salad mixture. Mix the oil and lemon juice and sprinkle over the top. Serve at once.

serves 2

baked aubergines with peppers, quinoa and broccoli salsa

Baby peppers and long-slim Italian peppers seem to have the most intense flavours when baked.

ingredients

2 medium aubergines, cut in half lengthways
a little cold-pressed mixed seed oil
4 small whole red or orange sweet peppers
100g (3½ oz) hummus
10–12 black olives, pitted and chopped
2–3 spring onions, trimmed and chopped
1 tablespoon freshly chopped or 1 teaspoon dried tarragon
100g (3½ oz) quinoa

BROCCOLI SALSA
100g (3½ oz) broccoli head, broken into small florets
1 small red or orange pepper, seeded and finely chopped
1 spring onion, trimmed and chopped
1cm (½ in) fresh root ginger, peeled and grated
juice of 1 lime
1 teaspoon cold-pressed mixed seed oil

method

1 Set the oven to 200°C/400°F/Gas 6.

2 Cut a criss-cross pattern on the cut surface of the aubergines and brush all over with a little mixed seed oil. Place on a baking tray, cut side down, with the peppers and bake for about 25–30 minutes or until the vegetables are almost cooked through.

3 Mix the hummus with the olives, spring onions and tarragon and keep on one side.

4 After 30 minutes' cooking, turn the aubergines over, spread with the hummus mixture and return to the oven for another 5–10 minutes until fully cooked.

5 Meanwhile cook the quinoa as directed on page 37. Mix all the Broccoli Salsa ingredients together just before serving and hand round with the baked vegetables and quinoa.

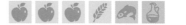 serves 2

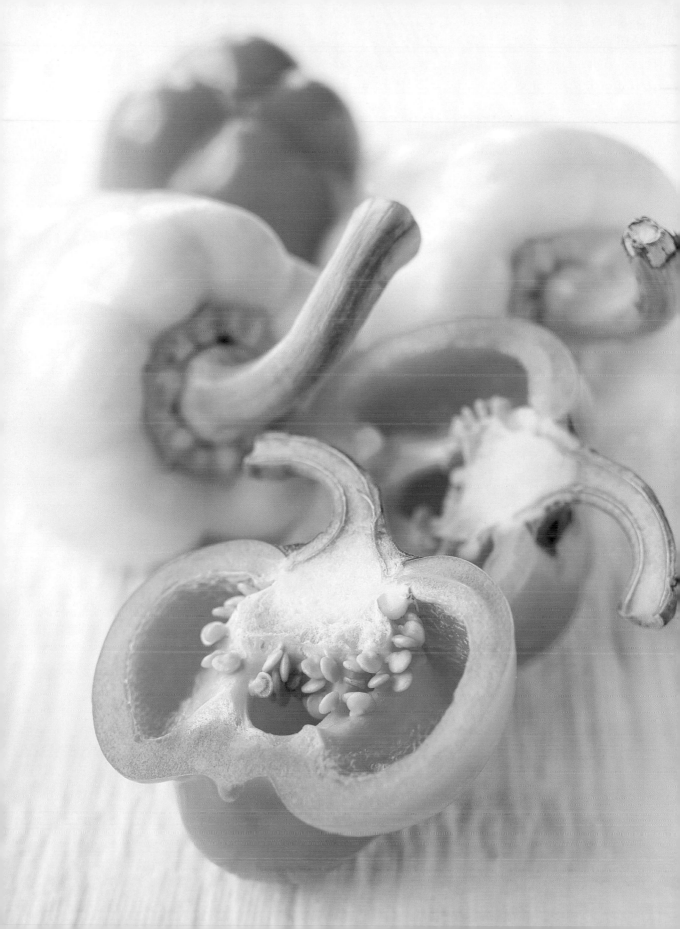

red mullet baked in a paper case

This is one of the ways in which red mullet is cooked in the South of France and you really cannot add too much garlic! If you prefer fresh herbs, use at least double the quantities (maybe a little more). Serve some boiled potatoes on the side.

ingredients
a little extra-virgin olive oil
2–3 shallots, peeled and finely sliced
2–6 red mullet (depending on size), cleaned
3–4 tomatoes, skinned, seeded and chopped
2–3 cloves garlic, peeled and crushed
¼ teaspoon fennel seeds, crushed in a mortar
¼ teaspoon dried thyme
a pinch of dried rosemary
freshly ground black pepper (to taste)
2 tablespoons freshly chopped parsley

method
1 Preheat the oven to 180°C/350°F/Gas 4 and prepare two large double squares of baking parchment. Lightly brush the top layers with olive oil.

2 Place the shallots in the cavities of the fish and place half the fish on each square of prepared parchment. Mix all the remaining ingredients together, except the parsley, and spoon over the fish.

3 Carefully close up each parcel, folding the edges over so that no steam can escape. Place on a baking tray and bake for 20–25 minutes for small fish and 25–30 minutes for larger fish. Serve in the paper cases so that each person can unwrap their own portion.

4 Put the chopped parsley in a separate dish for each person to sprinkle over their fish as they unwrap it.

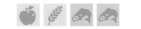 serves 2

chickpea crumble with leafy avocado salad

Flavour and texture are all-important in this easily prepared, highly nutritious, main-course dish.

ingredients

1 small onion, peeled and chopped
1 stick celery, chopped
½ small red pepper, chopped
2 carrots, peeled and chopped
1 teaspoon extra-virgin olive oil

a little vegetable stock or water
1 x 200g (7oz) can tomatoes
175g (6oz) canned chickpeas,
 drained
a pinch of ground cumin

CRUMBLE
100g (3½ oz) wholemeal flour or brown rice flour
25g (1oz) oatflakes
1 tablespoon pumpkin seeds
3 tablespoons cold-pressed seed oil

LEAFY AVOCADO SALAD
mixed salad leaves
1 small or ½ large avocado, peeled, pitted and chopped

DRESSING
3 dessertspoons cold-pressed mixed seed oil
1 dessertspoon cider vinegar

method

1 Set the oven to 190°C/375°F/Gas 5. Steam-fry the onion, celery, red pepper and carrots in the olive oil with a little stock or water for about 5 minutes until the carrots begin to soften. Add the tomatoes, chickpeas and cumin and bring to the boil. Cover and simmer for 10–15 minutes.

2 Meanwhile, mix the dry Crumble ingredients in a bowl and rub in the seed oil until the mixture resembles breadcrumbs.

3 Pour the chickpea mixture into an ovenproof dish about 15cm (6 in) in diameter and sprinkle the Crumble over the top. Place in the oven and bake for 30 minutes.

4 For the Leafy Avocado Salad, place the salad leaves in two small bowls and top with the chopped avocado. Mix the Dressing ingredients in a cup and sprinkle over the salads. Serve with the Chickpea Crumble.

 serves 2

vegetable parcels with chilli sauce and kiwi salsa

It is worth making the effort to have a go at these attractive little parcels when you are entertaining. The quantities given here make 12 parcels or enough for four people.

ingredients

75g (3oz) green or brown whole lentils
350ml (11fl oz) vegetable stock
75g (3oz) quinoa
175g (6oz) carrots, peeled and chopped
1 medium onion, peeled and chopped
2–3 sticks celery, sliced
125g (4½ oz) canned or cooked sweetcorn kernels
15g (½ oz) fresh coriander
15g (½ oz) fresh parsley
freshly ground black pepper (to taste)
24 squares filo pastry, approximately 20–22cm (8–9 in square)
extra-virgin olive oil

CHILLI SAUCE
4 large ripe tomatoes, peeled, or 1 x 200g (7oz) can tomatoes
2 cloves garlic, peeled and crushed
2 fresh red chillies, seeded and finely chopped
a pinch of dried thyme

KIWI SALSA
2 kiwi fruit, peeled and diced
1 tomato, diced
1 small fresh red chilli, seeded and finely chopped
4 spring onions, trimmed and finely chopped
a pinch of ground cumin
juice of ½ lemon

method

1 Place the lentils and stock in a saucepan. Cover and cook for 10 minutes. Add the quinoa and return to the boil. Cover and cook for a further 15–20 minutes until the lentils and quinoa are cooked and all the liquid has evaporated.

2 Meanwhile, place the chopped and sliced vegetables in a steamer for 5 minutes over boiling water to soften them. Chop again and place in a large mixing bowl. Stir in the sweetcorn, herbs and pepper and finally the cooked lentils and quinoa. Mix well together.

3 Set the oven to 200°C/400°F/Gas 6.

4 Brush the squares of filo pastry with oil and arrange in piles of three. Place a heaped table-spoon of the vegetable mixture on each one, gather up into a money bag parcel and secure with a length of cotton. Place on a baking tray and bake for 15–20 minutes until well browned. (Remove the cotton before serving.)

5 Chop the tomatoes very finely and place in a saucepan with all the remaining sauce ingredients. Bring to the boil and cook over a medium heat, stirring from time to time, until the mixture thickens. Serve with the Vegetable Parcels.

6 Place all the Kiwi Salsa ingredients in a bowl and mix well. Leave to stand until required.

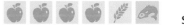 serves 4

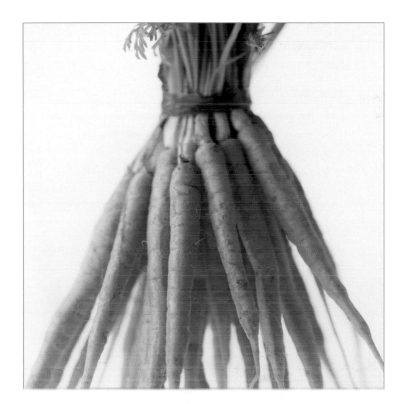

stuffed squash with watercress salad

You could use almost any type of squash for this recipe but the buttery red flesh of the pear-shaped butternut has a particularly good texture and flavour.

ingredients

1 butternut squash, approximately 750g (1lb 10oz)

a little extra-virgin olive oil or cold-pressed mixed seed oil

100g (3½ oz) quinoa

150ml (5fl oz) vegetable stock

1 small red pepper, seeded and cut into small pieces

175g (6oz) sweetcorn kernels

2 tablespoons sunflower seeds

100g (3½ oz) grated cheese (optional)

a pinch of freshly grated nutmeg

WATERCRESS SALAD

½ bunch watercress

1 Little Gem lettuce

5cm (2in) length cucumber, sliced

a handful of alfalfa sprouts

DRESSING

25ml (1fl oz) cold-pressed mixed seed oil

3 tablespoons low-fat natural live yoghurt

1 small tomato

1 teaspoon cider vinegar

1 clove garlic, peeled and crushed

a spring onion, chopped

a large sprig of fresh basil, chopped

a pinch each of paprika, black pepper and mustard powder

method

1 Preheat the oven to 200°C/400°F/Gas 6.

2 Cut the butternut squash in half and place, flesh side up, on a baking tray. Drizzle with a little oil and bake for about 45 minutes until tender.

3 Cook the quinoa in the vegetable stock for 15 minutes until all the water has evaporated and the quinoa is tender. Gently cook the pepper in a little more oil until it has softened.

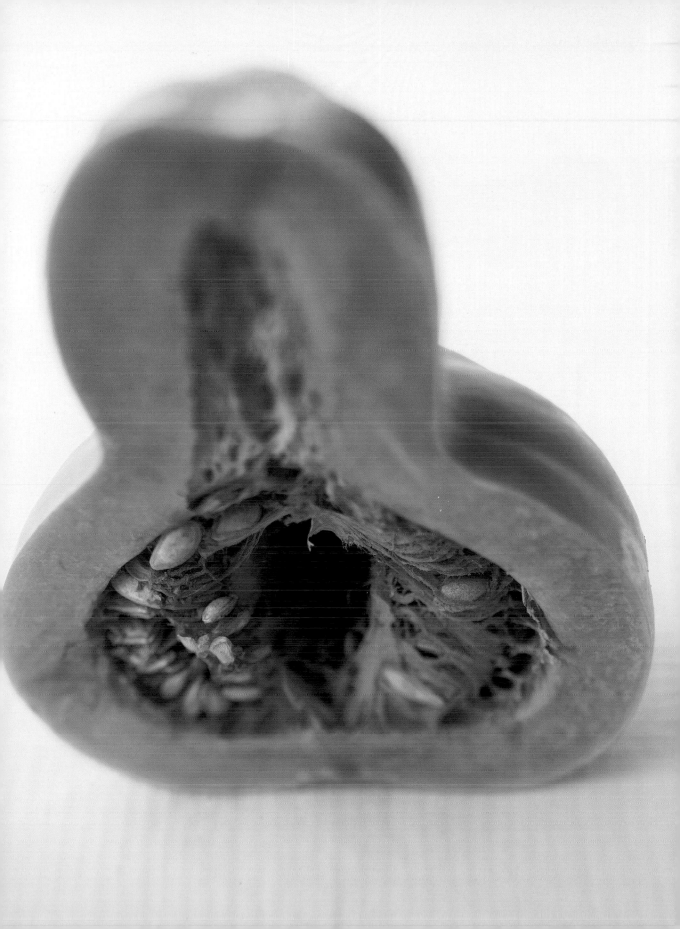

4 When the squash is cooked, remove the seeds and spoon out the flesh, taking care not to damage the skin. Mix with the quinoa, red pepper, sweetcorn, sunflower seeds, cheese and nutmeg. Spoon this back into the skins and return to the oven for a further 10–15 minutes.

5 For the Watercress Salad, start by placing all the Dressing ingredients in a blender and process until well mixed. The mixture will go slightly creamy.

6 Mix all the Watercress Salad ingredients together in a bowl, toss with the Dressing and serve at once with the Butternut Squash.

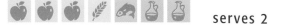 serves 2

potato, coriander and courgette pie

This mildly spiced dish needs a well-flavoured cheese for the best effect.

ingredients

2½–3 tablespoons chopped fresh coriander
150g (5½ oz) Spenwood or Pecorino ewe's milk cheese, grated
1 clove garlic, peeled and finely chopped
1cm (½ in) fresh root ginger, peeled and finely chopped
350g (12oz) potatoes, peeled and thinly sliced
175g (6oz) courgettes, thinly sliced
1 large onion, peeled and thinly sliced
75ml (3fl oz) white wine or vegetable stock

method

1 Set the oven to 190°C/375°F/Gas 5.

2 Mix the coriander, cheese, garlic and ginger in a bowl.

3 Line a dish with half the potatoes and cover with half the courgettes and then half the sliced onion. Next, spoon on half the cheese mixture. Continue with second layers of potato, courgette and onion, using up all that remain. Pour on the wine or stock and cover with foil.

4 Bake in the oven for an hour until a skewer finds the potato tender. Top with the remaining cheese mixture and finish off under the grill.

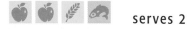 serves 2

desserts

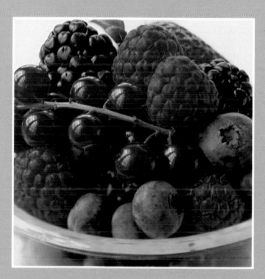

baked apples with seville orange marmalade

Seville orange marmalade gives a wonderfully tangy flavour to baked apples.

ingredients
2 large Bramley cooking apples
6–8 dates, pitted
1 tablespoon Seville orange marmalade
2 teaspoons ground almonds, hazelnuts or sunflower seeds
4 tablespoons cloudy apple juice

method **1** Preheat the oven to 220°C/425°F/Gas 7.

2 Wash and core the apples. Cut round the centre of each apple to stop them splitting during cooking. Stuff with the dates, marmalade, ground nuts or seeds and place in an ovenproof dish.

3 Pour on the apple juice and bake for about 45 minutes until the apple is cooked through.

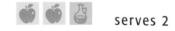 serves 2

winter fruit salad

Squeeze the oranges before you prepare the fruit. Each piece of fruit can then go straight into the juice. This helps to cut down on vitamin loss and discoloration.

ingredients
juice of 2 oranges
1 small green-skinned apple, cored and diced
1 small red-skinned apple, cored and diced
1 kiwi fruit, peeled and diced
6 kumquats, sliced
50g (2oz) no-soak dried apricots, halved

method **1** Pour the orange juice into a bowl and add all the remaining ingredients as you prepare them.

2 Toss together and serve at once.

 serves 2

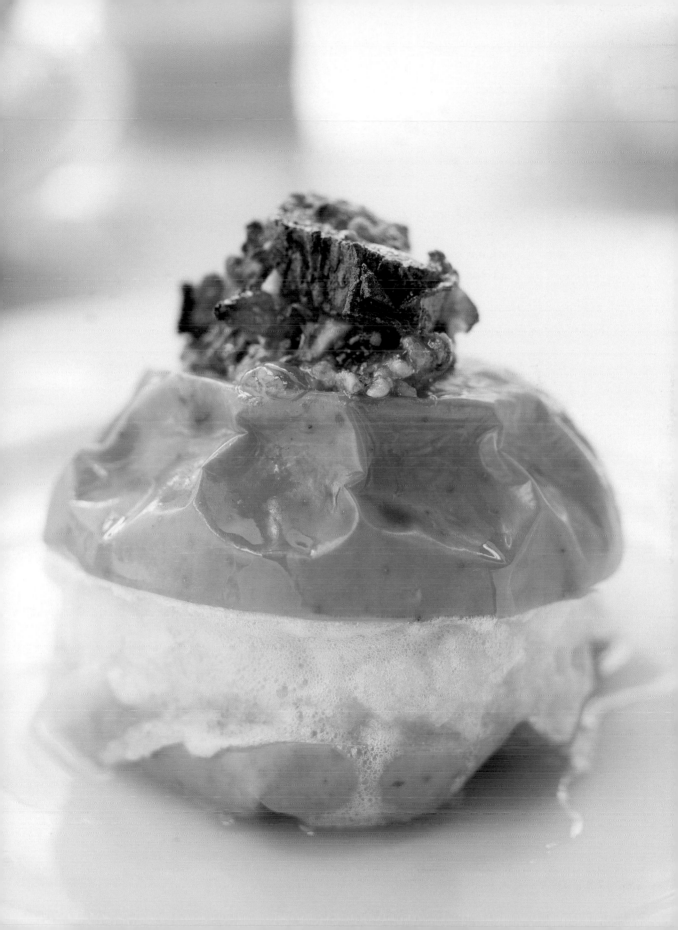

papaya cups with strawberries and lime

I first had this refreshing combination of fruits in Barbados, where it was served for break-fast. There is, of course, no reason why you should not do the same but the mixture does make an excellent dessert.

ingredients

1 large ripe papaya
juice of 1 lime

100g (3½ oz) strawberries
a few sprigs of fresh mint

method

1 Cut the papaya in half lengthways and scoop out all the seeds with a sharp teaspoon. Squeeze the lime and pour half the juice into each papaya half.

2 Quickly wash and hull the strawberries and cut in half. Pile into the papaya cups and serve garnished with the sprigs of fresh mint.

serves 2

banana nut cream

This is really rather rich but it does make an excellent special-occasion dessert. Add chopped dates or no-soak apricots for a change.

ingredients

2 bananas
juice of ½ lemon
75g (3oz) Greek yoghurt
25g (1oz) chopped walnuts or pistachio nuts
15g (½ oz) chopped sunflower seeds
a little grated lemon zest

method

1 Mash the bananas with a fork and quickly mix with the lemon juice to prevent oxidation.

2 Stir in the yoghurt, nuts, seeds and lemon zest and spoon into two bowls. Serve at once.

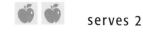

serves 2

raisin and vanilla tofucake

Tofucake is our name for a cheesecake made with tofu. There are no wheat or milk products in the cake but it does include eggs. It makes a splendid dessert or you could serve it with tea or coffee.

Take care when cutting, and serve with a fork as the base tends to be rather crumbly.

ingredients

50g (2oz) cornflakes
50g (2oz) cashew nuts
1 ½ tablespoons cold-pressed mixed seed oil
200g (7oz) firm tofu
2–3 tablespoons honey (to taste)
2 teaspoons vanilla essence
grated zest of 1 orange
4 eggs, separated
50g (2oz) brown rice flour
1 teaspoon baking powder
50g (2oz) raisins or sultanas

method

1 Preheat the oven to 180°C/350°F/Gas 4 and grease a 20cm (8 in) loose-based sandwich cake tin.

2 Grind the cornflakes and nuts in a food processor until quite fine and mix with the seed oil. Press this mixture into the base of the prepared cake tin and smooth over with the back of a spoon. Place in the oven and bake for 5–6 minutes.

3 Meanwhile, process the tofu with the honey, vanilla, orange zest and egg yolks in a food processor. Spoon into a bowl and fold in the brown rice flour, baking powder and raisins.

4 In another bowl, whisk the egg whites until they are very stiff and fold 1 tablespoonful into the tofu mixture. Then fold in the rest and spoon over the baked base.

5 Return to the oven and bake for about 35 minutes, covering with foil after about 20–25 minutes to prevent over-browning. Remove the base from the ring but leave the cake to cool on the base before serving.

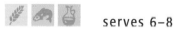 **serves 6–8**

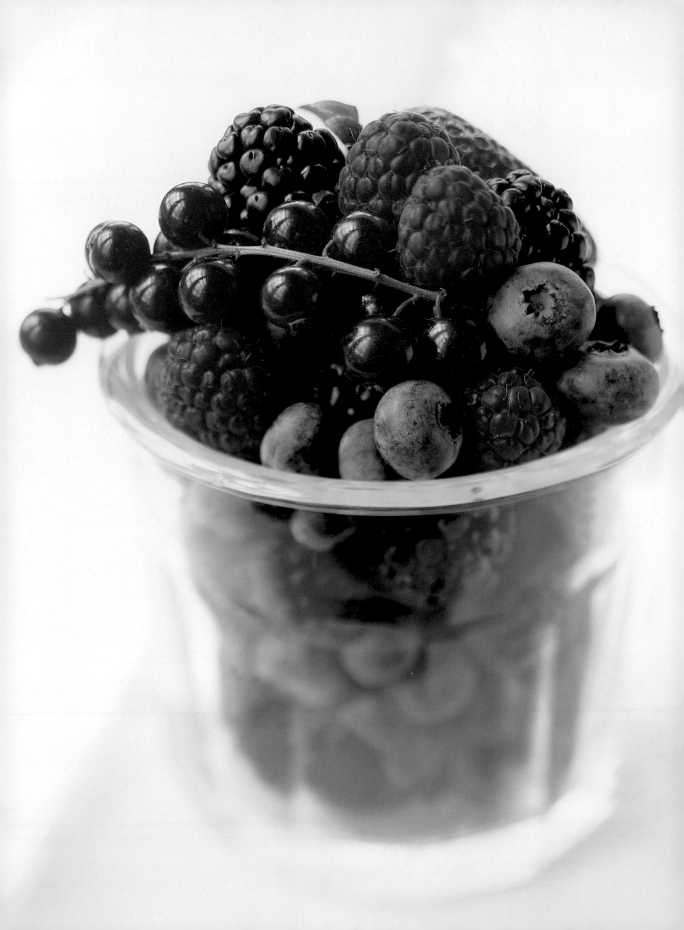

raspberry fool

Most berry fruits lend themselves to this simple treatment. Try blackberries, blackcurrants or blueberries. You can also use frozen fruits but the result will be much sloppier, as frozen berries do not hold their texture.

ingredients

150g (5½ oz) fresh raspberries, crushed with a fork
75g (3oz) low-fat fromage frais
a little honey (optional)
a few sprigs of fresh mint

method

1 Mix the raspberries, fromage frais and honey, if using, in a basin.

2 Spoon into two bowls and decorate with the sprigs of fresh mint to serve.

 serves 2

hunza apricots with cashew cream

This is quite a fiddly dish but it is worth making the effort for its delicious combination of flavours. Hunza apricots are smaller than ordinary ones and come with their stone in place. They are more nutritious than ordinary ones and you can buy them in healthfood shops.

ingredients

100g (3½ oz) Hunza apricots
25–40g (1–1½ oz) whole hazelnuts
50g (2oz) cashew nuts

method

1 Place the apricots in a bowl, cover with boiling water and leave to stand overnight to soften.

2 When the apricots are soft, carefully remove each apricot stone and replace with a whole hazelnut. Arrange the stuffed apricots in two bowls.

3 Grind the cashew nuts in a blender and process until very fine. Transfer to a basin and slowly blend in 50ml (2fl oz) water to make a smooth cream. Pour over the stuffed apricots and serve.

 serves 2

date and orange flan

This is another year-round dessert. Use dried dates in the winter and fresh ones in the summer. You may find that you do not need so much honey to bind the fresh date mixture.

ingredients
75g (3oz) dried dates, pitted and chopped
50g (2oz) ground almonds
1 tablespoon honey
4 tablespoons Greek yoghurt
grated zest of ½ orange
2 oranges, peeled and with zest removed and sliced separately

method **1** Chop the dates even further, in a food processor if possible. Mix in the almonds and honey and press the mixture into the base of a 15cm (6 in) flan tin. Place in the fridge and leave for at least an hour or until required.

2 Remove the flan base from the tin. Mix the yoghurt and orange zest and spread over the base. Arrange the orange slices on the top and serve.

 serves 2

apricot and almond dessert

Here's a simple but effective way to serve any kind of dried fruit. We have chosen Hunza apricots for their intense flavour and high iron and vitamin content.

ingredients
150g (5½ oz) Hunza apricots
2 tablespoons flaked almonds
150g (5½ oz) Greek yoghurt or thick-set soya yoghurt
a pinch of ground cinnamon

method **1** Place the apricots in a bowl, cover with boiling water and leave to stand overnight. When soft, carefully remove the stones.

2 Toast the flaked almonds in a dry frying pan over a medium heat. Stir regularly to prevent the nuts burning. Leave to cool and then crush lightly to break up the flakes.

3 Place the apricots in two large wine glasses, retaining two whole ones for decoration. Spoon in the yoghurt and sprinkle with cinnamon. Finally, add the toasted nuts and the retained apricots. Place in the fridge to chill for an hour or so before serving.

serves 2

baked cardamom custards

Make the dessert course your protein course with this creamy custard with a touch of the East. Start the meal with Gazpacho (see page 100) in summer or Celery and Apple Soup (see page 104) in the winter. Then serve Giambotta with Mixed Green Vegetables (see page 166) or Stuffed Squash with Watercress Salad (see page 192).

ingredients

300ml (10fl oz) skimmed, soya or rice milk
1 tablespoon clear honey
2 small eggs, beaten
seeds from 3 cardamom pods, crushed

method   **1** Set the oven to 150°C/300°F/Gas 8.

2 Beat the milk and honey into the eggs and sprinkle in the crushed seeds. Pour the mixture into two 10cm (4in) ramekins and place these in turn in a baking tin.

3 Pour very hot water into the baking tin to come about one-third of the way up the ramekins. Then bake for about an hour until a knife comes out clean when inserted in the centre.

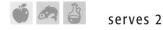

serves 2

dried fruit compôte with orange

Any mix of dried fruits can be used in this compôte – in fact, the wider the variety, the better! You should be able to find apples, apricots, peaches or nectarines, prunes, Lexia raisins, bananas, cherries, mangoes and figs.

ingredients

175g (6oz) mixed dried fruits
juice and zest of 1 large orange

method

1 Place the dried fruits in a bowl and cover with boiling water. Leave to stand for 2 hours. (If there are any ready-to-use fruits in the mix leave them on one side until later.)

2 Drain the fruits, place them in a saucepan with a little fresh water and bring to the boil. Cover and cook for 5 minutes (or until the toughest fruit is tender) and leave to cool.

3 Add any no-cook fruit and stir in the orange juice and zest. Chill until required.

 serves 2

sesame orange segments with cherries

Look for unwaxed organic oranges when you want to eat the zest.

ingredients

2 oranges
1 tablespoon sesame seeds
1 tablespoon wheatgerm

low-fat natural live yoghurt
12 fresh cherries

method

1 Grate the zest from one of the oranges and mix with the sesame seeds and wheatgerm. Then peel and segment both oranges, removing any excess pith.

2 Dip each segment in yoghurt and coat with the sesame mixture. Arrange on two plates with the cherries.

 serves 2

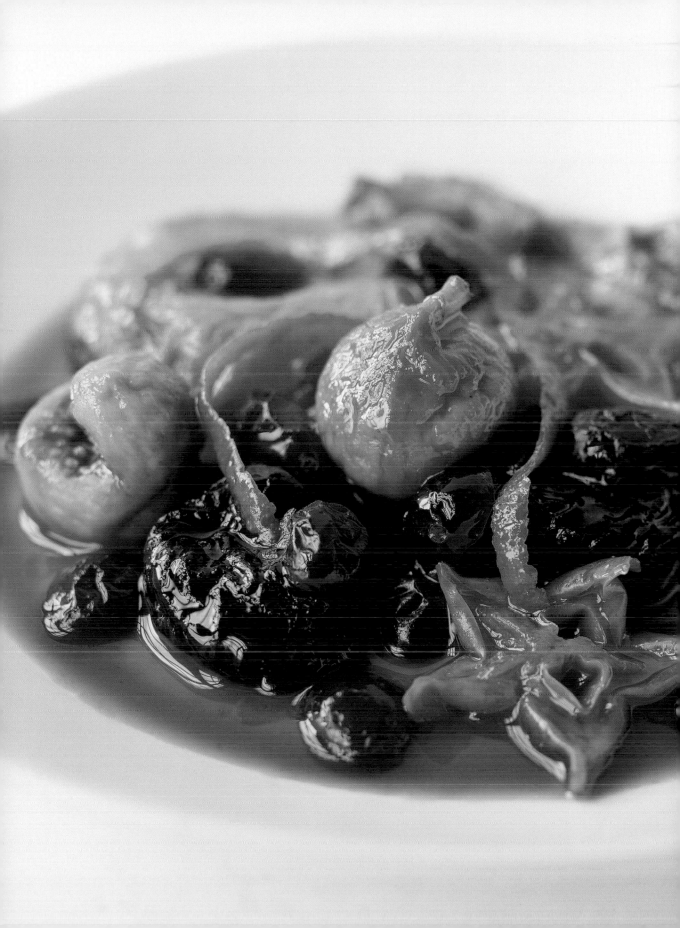

fruit crumble

This crumble topping is everyone's favourite and almost everyone can eat it. It is wheat-, fat-, dairy- and egg-free. Here it is served with apple but you can use it on all your favourite fruit bases.

ingredients

1 large cooking apple, peeled, cored and diced
lemon juice
1 tablespoon raisins
a little grated lemon zest

TOPPING
50g (2oz) rice or millet flakes
25g (1oz) flaked almonds, crushed
25g (1oz) brown rice flour
2–3 tablespoons hot brown rice syrup or honey

method

1 Set the oven to 190°C/375°F/Gas 5.

2 Prepare the apple and drop the pieces into a bowl of water with a little lemon juice in. Drain and transfer to a saucepan. Heat through until the apples being to sizzle a bit but do not cook them.

3 To make the Topping, mix the flakes, almonds and rice flour in a bowl. Spoon on the heated syrup or honey and stir in to bind the mixture. You may need to work it in with your hands.

4 Transfer the hot apples to an ovenproof dish and mix with the raisins and lemon zest. Sprinkle the prepared Topping evenly over the apples. Place in the oven and bake for about 25 minutes. Do not allow the Topping to brown too much or you will find it is too hard.

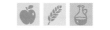 **serves 2**

sweet potato and ginger soufflé

Sweet potatoes are so sweet in themselves that you do not need to add any sugar to this deliciously fluffy dessert. It is possible to make a small soufflé but it makes such a good dinner party dessert that we have given quantities for four people.

ingredients

1 large or 2 sweet potatoes, approximately 500g (1lb 2oz)
75ml (3fl oz) canned coconut milk
2 teaspoons freshly grated fresh root ginger
1 teaspoon grated lemon zest
½ teaspoon baking powder
3 eggs, well beaten
1 tablespoon desiccated coconut

method

1 Preheat the oven to 190°C/375°F/Gas 5 and grease a small 20cm (8 in) soufflé dish.

2 Place the sweet potatoes in the oven and bake for about an hour until they are cooked through and soft. Scrape the flesh from the skins and place in a bowl.

3 Stir in the coconut milk, ginger, lemon zest and baking powder. Fold in the beaten eggs, pour into the prepared soufflé dish and sprinkle the top with the coconut.

4 Bake for about 40–45 minutes, until the soufflé starts to come away from the sides of the dish and a skewer through the centre comes out clean. Serve at once.

 serves 4

baked raisin and rice pudding

Rice pudding used to be the nursery pudding and a good filling dessert for all the family. Today it has rather fallen from grace, and pudding (or short-grain) rice is quite difficult to find in smaller supermarkets. Here's a well flavoured version of the old favourite.

ingredients

25g (1oz) pudding rice
250ml (9fl oz) milk
25g (1oz) raisins
ground nutmeg

method

1 Preheat the oven to 150°C/300°F/Gas 2 and grease a small ovenproof dish.

2 Place the rice, milk and raisins in the prepared dish and sprinkle with nutmeg. Place in the oven and bake for 1½–2 hours, depending on how thick you like your rice pudding to be.

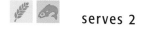 **serves 2**

pears in blackcurrant coulis

This is very much an all-year-round recipe, as you can use frozen blackcurrants just as easily as fresh ones. You could also use raspberries, tayberries or loganberries.

ingredients

150g (5½oz) blackcurrants
1 tablespoon Crème de Cassis (optional)
a little runny honey (to taste)
2 very ripe pears, peeled
a few sprigs of mint

method

1 Reserve a few whole blackcurrants and rub the rest through a sieve, extracting as much pulp as possible. This might be easier if you heat the fruit a little, though you will reduce the vitamin content slightly. Discard the pips and skins and mix the purée with the liqueur, and the honey if using.

2 Place the peeled pears on individual plates and pour the blackcurrant purée over the top. Decorate with the reserved berries and the sprigs of mint. Serve at once.

serves 2

rhubarb and blackcurrant pie

The ground almonds form a kind of crust on top of the fruit in this easy-to-make hot dessert. You can use any kind of fresh or frozen berries.

ingredients

125g (4½oz) rhubarb, trimmed and cut into small pieces
50g (2oz) low-fat soft cheese
1 dessertspoon runny honey
125g (4½oz) blackcurrants
25–40g (1–1½oz) ground almonds

method

1 Place the rhubarb in two small heatproof dishes and sprinkle with 4 teaspoons water. Cover with foil and bake for about 15 minutes.

2 Mix the cheese and honey to make a thick cream. Remove the foil from the rhubarb and add the blackcurrants. Spread on the cheese and honey mixture.

3 Place under a hot grill and cook for about 2–3 minutes. Sprinkle with the ground almonds and return to the grill. Cook for another 1–2 minutes until golden brown.

serves 2

christmas pudding

This wonderfully aromatic Christmas Pudding is very light and has everyone coming back for more! Serve with natural yoghurt, or a mixture of yoghurt and Cashew Cream (see page 201).

This quantity makes one large pudding, which will serve eight, or two smaller puddings.

ingredients

50g (2oz) ground almonds

75g (3oz) fresh wholemeal or rye breadcrumbs

75g (3oz) unsalted butter, cut into pieces

225g (8oz) Lexia raisins

225g (8oz) sultanas

1 orange, scrubbed, sliced and chopped

juice and grated zest of 1 lemon

1 medium Bramley cooking apple, cored and grated

2 eggs, beaten

3 tablespoons brandy

1 tablespoon soya milk

¼ teaspoon grated nutmeg

¼ teaspoon ground cinnamon

¼ teaspoon mixed spice

method

1 Place the ground almonds and breadcrumbs in a bowl with the butter. Then rub the butter into the dry ingredients until the mixture resembles breadcrumbs.

2 Stir in the raisins, sultanas and orange pieces. Add the lemon and apple. Mix the eggs with the brandy and milk and stir into the mixture with the spices.

3 Spoon the mixture into one large or two small pudding basins and cover with greaseproof paper and foil. Tie down tightly and steam for 4 hours. Steam for a further hour before serving.

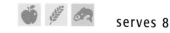 **serves 8**

drinks

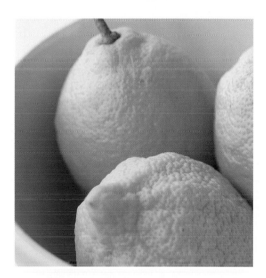

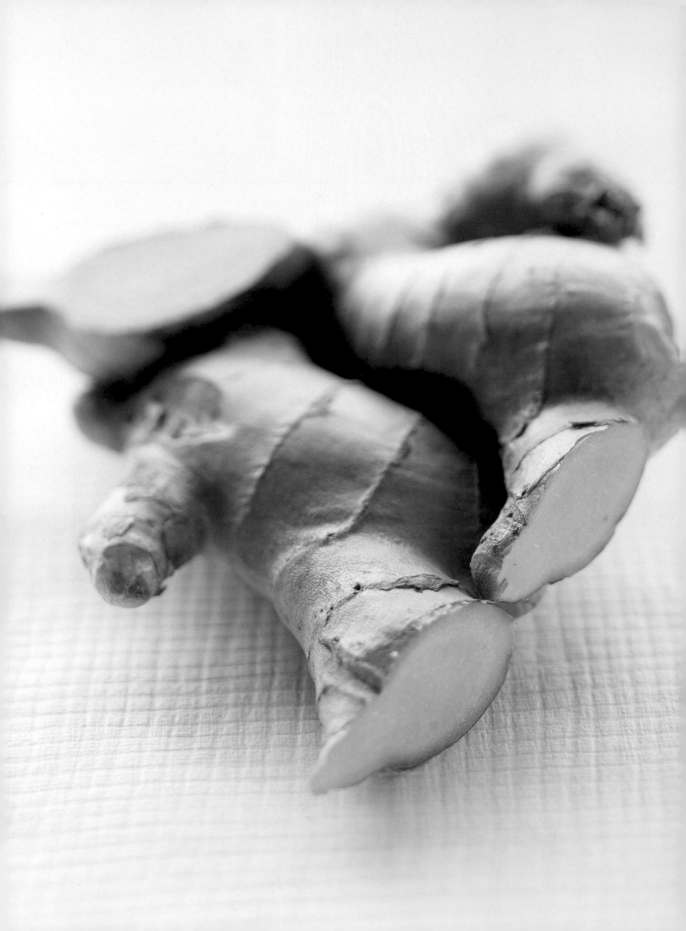

lemon ginger punch

This is such an easy drink to make that we often serve it in place of fruit teas and other infusions. It is wonderful for combating colds and stomach upsets.

Infuse the ginger and cinnamon at least twice or use larger quantities of water and drink later.

ingredients

a 2.5cm (1in) piece fresh ginger, scrubbed
1 stick cinnamon
juice of 1 lemon
a little honey (optional)

method

1 Slice the ginger and place in a mug with the cinnamon stick. Fill up the mug with boiling water. Infuse until the mixture is cool enough to drink.

2 Strain and stir in the lemon juice, and honey if using.

serves 1

lime and apple drink

Here's another simpler infusion drink – with fresh lime juice for added flavour.

ingredients

400ml (14fl oz) sugar-free apple juice
juice of 2 fresh limes
0.5cm (½in) thick slice of fresh ginger, peeled
2 sprigs fresh mint
1 small apple, cored and sliced

method

1 Mix the juices and add the slice of fresh ginger to infuse. Leave to cool in the fridge until required.

2 Serve with a sprig of mint and a few slices of fresh apple in each glass.

serves 2

watermelon whizz

Watermelons are rich in beta-carotene and vitamin C and their seeds also contain valuable quantities of essential fats, vitamin E, zinc and selenium. However, their seeds can be difficult to chew. The answer is to blend them with the flesh to create an incredibly immune-boosting drink.

ingredients   1 large chunk of watermelon per person

method   **1** Remove the skin and place each chunk of watermelon in a blender with all the seeds in place. Blend until smooth and frothy and serve at once.

 serves 2

berry juice cocktail

There is an ever-increasing variety of ready-made fruit and berry juices available and you can easily mix and match them to make some really interesting drinks. Choose those with no added sugar and add some water to dilute the natural fruit sugars.

Alternatively, you can make your own mixtures with a good apple juice base. One of the best is English apple juice made with fresh crushed fruit and no concentrates. My favourite blend is with raspberries.

ingredients   300ml (10fl oz) apple juice
225g (8oz) fresh berries, e.g. blueberries, blackberries, raspberries or
    strawberries (or a mixture of some of these)
crushed ice

method   **1** Put the apple juice in a blender and add the fruit. Whizz up and add the crushed ice. Serve at once.

 serves 2

hot blackcurrant cordial

Berry fruits are great immune-boosters and Hot Blackcurrant Cordial is really good for colds and sore throats. You can also use this simple method to produce hot berry cordials of all kinds.

Measure the fruit by volume, rather than by weight, to get the right ratio of water to fruit.

ingredients

1 cup or 200g (7oz) blackcurrants
honey (to taste)

method

1 Simmer the blackcurrants in 2 cups or 400ml (14fl oz) water for 10 minutes.

2 Strain, pressing through as much of the juice as possible. Add honey to taste.

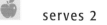

serves 2

ginger and apple blender drink

Everyone loves the tangy flavour and fluffy texture of this simple blender drink. Try it with pears instead of apples for a change.

ingredients

2 lumps stem ginger in honey, with 2 teaspoons of the juice
2 small apples, cored
300ml (10fl oz) sugar-free apple juice
juice of ½ lemon
ice cubes

method

1 Place all the ingredients, except the ice, in a blender and process until smooth. Serve at once with ice cubes. (If the mixture is left to stand, bits of apple and ginger will float to the top.)

serves 2

fruit shakes

There is no comparison between the flavour of a home-made fruit shake and the packet variety. Nor is there any comparison between the nutritional value of the two! Here are some ideas for delicious fruit shake combinations, each making one serving.

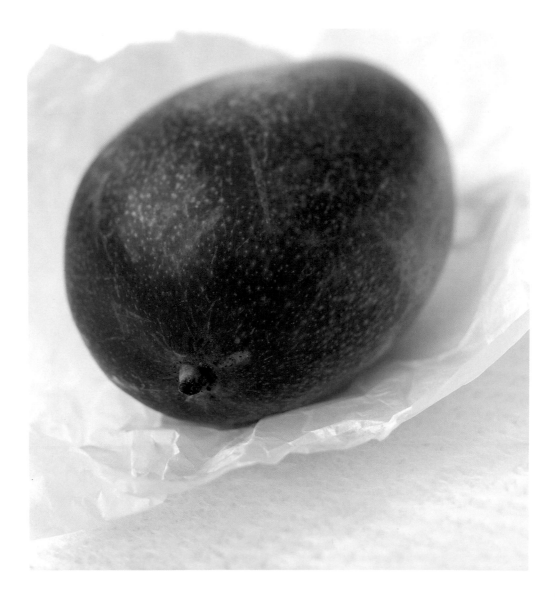

mango and banana dream

ingredients

1 small banana
1 small mango
25g (1oz) low-fat natural live yoghurt
150–200ml (5–7fl oz) sugar-free apple juice (to taste)
ice cubes

method

1 Peel the banana and peel and stone the mango and place the flesh of both fruits in a blender. Add the yoghurt and process until smooth.

2 Next, add sufficient apple juice to give the required texture. Serve with ice cubes.

 serves 2

pear and raspberry yoghurt shake

Some popular variations on this theme include banana and kiwi fruit or gooseberries and strawberries.

ingredients

150g (5½oz) low-fat natural live yoghurt
½ teaspoon honey (optional)
200g (7oz) raspberries
1 pear, peeled and cored
1 dessertspoon ground flax and pumpkin seeds
75–100ml (3–4fl oz) skimmed, soya or rice milk

method

1 Place all the ingredients, except the milk, in a blender and whizz to a smooth cream. Add milk to achieve the consistency you prefer.

serves 2

sesame and papaya shake

The sesame seeds add essential fatty acids to this tropical shake.

ingredients

2 tablespoons sesame seeds *or* 1 tablespoon sesame seeds and 1 tablespoon
sunflower seeds
1 medium-sized papaya
juice of 1 orange
300ml (10fl oz) soya milk
a little grated orange rind (optional)

method

1 Soak the seeds overnight in 2 tablespoons water.

2 In the morning, process in a blender, then add the fruit and process again.

3 Top up with the orange juice and soya milk to give your desired consistency and serve. Add a little grated orange rind, if liked.

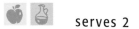

serves 2

mixed fruit and seed shake

If you find the Omega Drink on page 219 a little difficult to take, try this version (which is mixed with fresh fruit) and simply drink more of it to make up the quantity of essential fatty acids.

ingredients

2 teaspoons linseeds
2 teaspoons sunflower seeds
1 small banana, peeled
1 kiwi fruit, skin removed
2 apricots (or 1 peach or nectarine or a small pear), peeled and pitted or
cored
25g (1oz) low-fat natural live yoghurt
100–150ml (4–5fl oz) rice milk or soya milk

method   **1** Grind the seeds and prepare the fruit.

2 Place the seeds and fruit in a blender with the yoghurt and half the milk. Blend until thick and smooth.

3 Add the remaining milk to taste and chill before serving.

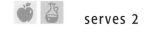 **serves 2**

omega drink

You may not think that this exceedingly nutritious drink is going to taste very good, but everyone who tries it is very pleasantly surprised!

ingredients

    2 tablespoons brown linseed or flax seeds
    1 tablespoon sunflower seeds
    1 small piece of fresh ginger (to taste), peeled and chopped
    150ml (5fl oz) sugar-free apple juice
    1 teaspoon lecithin granules (optional)

method   **1** Soak the seeds overnight in 100ml (4fl oz) water.

2 The next day, put the soaked seeds and their water in a blender. Add all the other ingredients and blend until thick and creamy.

3 Add a little more water if you prefer a thinner mixture. Pour into a glass and serve. Drink at once, before the mixture begins to settle and separate.

serves 2

Useful Addresses

Essential Oil Blends containing a combination of cold-pressed seed oils are becoming more widely available. One of the best is Udo's Choice, distributed by Savant Distribution, Quarry House, Clayton Wood Close, Leeds LS16 6QA. Tel: 08450 60 60 70 or visit www.savant-health.com.

The Institute for Optimum Nutrition (ION) offers a three-year foundation degree course in nutritional therapy that includes training in the optimum nutrition approach to mental health. There is a clinic, a list of nutrition practitioners across the UK, an information service and a quarterly journal – *Optimum Nutrition*. Contact ION at Avalon House, 72 Lower Mortlake Road, Richmond TW9 2JY. Tel: 0208 6147 7800 or visit www.ion.ac.uk. To find a nutritional therapist near you who we recommend, visit www.patrickholford.com and click on 'Advice' and then 'Find a nutritionist'.

Totally Nourish offers a wide range of health products, including supplements. Visit www.totallynourish.com. Tel: 0800 085 7749.

Low Sodium Sea Salt, high in magnesium, potassium and other beneficial trace minerals, and hence positively good for you, is available in Morrisons stores under the brand name Solo Sea Salt. Solo salt has been shown to lower blood pressure, rather than raise it. In case of difficulty, Solo is also available by mail-order from The Low Sodium Sea Salt Company Ltd, 101–103 Palace Road, Bromley, Kent BR1 3JZ. Tel: 0208 464 1665 or visit their website www.soloseasalt.com

Nutrition Consultation – to find a nutritional therapist in your area, visit www.patrickholford.com and select 'Advice' and then 'Find a nutritionist'. If there is no-one available nearby, you can get your ideal diet and supplement programme by completing the online 100% Health Programme.

Nutrition Assessment Online – you can have your own personal health and nutrition assessment online using the 100% Health Programme. Visit www.patrickholford.com and go to '100% Health Club'.

The Soil Association offers membership. For information, write to: The Soil Association, South Plaza, Marlborough Street, Bristol BS1 3NX. Tel: 0117 314 5000. Visit: www.soilassociation.org.